# Manage Your Pain: Transform Your Life

# Manage Your Pain: Transform Your Life

The ultimate guide to working with your body

Nikki Robinson

Holisticare Press

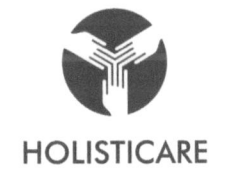

HOLISTICARE

Holisticare Press

*First published in 2023 by Holisticare Press*

*Copyright © Nikki Robinson 2023*

*The right of Nikki Robinson to be identified as the author of this work has been asserted by her in accordance with the Copyright, Designs and Patents Act 1988*

*ISBN 978-1-7393087-0-4*

*ISBN (ebook) 978-1-7393087-1-1*

*All rights reserved. No part of this publication, except for brief review, may be reproduced, stored or introduced into a retrieval system, or transmitted in any form, or by any means – electronic, mechanical, photocopying, recording, or otherwise – without the prior written permission of both the copyright owner and the publisher.*

**Illustrations:** *© Gabrielle Vickery Illustration*

**Photographs:** *© Sarah Padilha, Padilha Images and © Detheo Photography*

**Text design:** *Nikki Bull*

**Cover design:** *Lois Fordham*

# TABLE OF CONTENTS

FOREWORD – JOHN BARNES ..... 1

IMPORTANT NOTE ..... 2

INTRODUCTION ..... 3
- Why I wrote this book ..... 3
- How to use this book ..... 5
- Is this you? ..... 5

## CHAPTER 1 ..... 7
### YOUR FASCIA ..... 7
- The ideal body and what can go wrong ..... 7
- What is your fascia? ..... 9
- Biotensegrity ..... 11
- References ..... 14

## CHAPTER 2 ..... 15
### HOW YOUR BODY REACTS TO INJURY ..... 15
- Physical reaction ..... 15
- Reactions to perceived danger or stress ..... 17
- Emotional response ..... 18
- Falls ..... 22
- Concussion ..... 24
- References ..... 25

## CHAPTER 3 ..... 27
### COMMON SYMPTOMS ..... 27
- Pain ..... 27
- Tension ..... 30
- Inflammation ..... 32
- References ..... 33

## CHAPTER 4 ..... 35
### COMMON CONDITIONS ..... 35
- Auto-immune disorders ..... 35
- Back pain ..... 36
- Bursitis ..... 38
- Fibromyalgia ..... 38
- Frozen shoulder ..... 39
- Hypermobility ..... 40
- Incontinence ..... 40
- Joint pain and stiffness ..... 44
  - *Hand and wrist pain and stiffness* ..... 44
  - *Elbow pain and stiffness* ..... 44
  - *Shoulder pain and stiffness* ..... 45
  - *Knee pain and stiffness* ..... 46
  - *Hip pain and stiffness* ..... 46
- Joint replacements ..... 47
- Long Covid ..... 47
- Mental health conditions ..... 48
- Neck pain ..... 49

Neurological conditions ............ 50
Osteoarthritis ............................ 50
Plantar fasciitis ....................... 52
Repetitive strain injury .............. 52
Rotator cuff injury .................... 53
Scar tissue ............................... 53
Surgery .................................... 54
Tendonitis ................................ 55
References ............................... 56

# CHAPTER 5 .......... 57
## SIMPLE STEPS TO WORKING WITH YOUR BODY .................... 57

Drink enough water .................... 57
Breathe properly ........................ 59
Stretch ..................................... 63
Listen to your body ................... 65
Posture .................................... 68
References ............................... 69

# CHAPTER 6 .......... 71
## EVERYDAY WAYS TO HELP YOURSELF ............ 71

Lifting ...................................... 71
Gardening ................................ 73
Technology .............................. 75
Babies and children .................. 77

# CHAPTER 7 .......... 79
## TREATING YOURSELF .... 79

Feeling your body ...................... 80
How to treat yourself ................ 81
   *Using your hands* ............... 81
   *Using the contract/relax method* ...................... 81
   *Using a ball* ........................ 82
   *Using a foam roller* ............. 83
Things to remember .................. 84
How to help scars ..................... 84
How to help your neck and upper back ........................... 85
   *The front of your neck* .......... 85
   *Ball release for the back of your neck* ....................... 85
   *The side of your neck* .......... 86
How to help the middle of your back .............................. 87
   *Side stretch* ........................ 87
   *Diaphragm release with foam roller* .................. 87
How to help your lower back ..... 88
   *Back release using a ball* ..... 88
   *Back release in standing* ...... 89
   *Back release using a foam roller* .......................... 90
   *The Constructive Rest Position* ............................... 91
How to help your legs ............... 92
   *Releasing the front of your upper leg using a ball* .......... 92
   *Releasing the back of your upper leg* ..................... 93

*Releasing the backs of
your upper legs with
a foam roller.*........................ 94

*Releasing the tendon on
the outside of your upper
leg with a foam roller* .......... 94

*Seated contract / relax
exercise to release
your hips* .............................. 95

*Buttocks release* ................... 96

*Calf release using a ball*...... 97

*For tired legs* ....................... 98

How to help your arms ............... 98

*Elbow release*....................... 98

*Shoulder release* .................. 99

*Chest release*........................ 99

*Shoulder blade release* ...... 101

How to help your hands
and feet ..................................... 101

*Releasing your hand
using a ball* ........................ 101

*Finger pulls*........................ 102

*Release for the tops
of your feet*......................... 103

*Releasing your foot on
a ball* .................................. 104

*Foot on foot release*........... 104

How to help your head
and face..................................... 105

*Releasing your temples*...... 105

*Releasing your forehead*.... 106

*Sinus release* ...................... 107

*Hair pull*............................. 107

*Ear pulls*............................. 108

References ................................ 109

# CHAPTER 8 ......... 111
## MYOFASCIAL RELEASE.111

What is myofascial release?...... 111

What does it involve?............... 113

*Assessment* ......................... *113*

*Treatment* ........................... *114*

*Healing crisis*..................... *115*

*Unwinding* ......................... *116*

References ................................ 117

# CHAPTER 9 ......... 119
## PATIENT STORIES.......... 119

# CHAPTER 10 ....... 133
## ONGOING HELP............. 133

Holisticare................................ 133

The Let it Go Programme ........ 134

Freedom From Pain and
Tension – online programme.... 134

Mailing list................................ 135

Pain-Free Horse Riding............ 135

Get in touch .............................. 135

ACKNOWLEDGMENTS.. 137

BIBLIOGRAPHY ............ 139

GLOSSARY..................... 141

INDEX .............................. 145

> *Healing is a journey, not an event.*
>
> John F. Barnes

# FOREWORD – JOHN BARNES

I have had the honor and opportunity of knowing Nikki Robinson for a number of years through my myofascial release seminars. She is a highly intelligent, excellent therapist, who has combined her love of horses with her expertise in myofascial release.

I was an athlete when I was younger, and I fell with 300 pounds in a weightlifting contest which ruptured a disc in my lower back area. I tried every form of therapy including surgery to get better, nothing worked. There was a day when I realized that there's nobody going to help me, but me. Nobody wanted to get better more than I. I started to treat myself on my living room floor. Over time, I started to make a remarkable recovery. I then utilized these principles, which are totally different than other forms of traditional therapy, on my patients.

Science is verifying the principles of myofascial release that I have been teaching now for over 40 years. Fascia is an incredibly powerful connective tissue that connects and intersperses with every muscle, bone, nerve, organ, and cell in our body. When restricted, fascial restrictions can generate tensile forces of up to approximately 2,000 pounds per square inch of pressure. Crushing pressure! The important point here also is that fascial restrictions do not show up in any of the standard testing that is currently being offered for humans or animals; X-rays, CAT scans, blood work, etc. Therefore, fascial restrictions have been misdiagnosed for eons. A highly trained therapist, such as Nikki, can feel where the restrictions lie in a particular individual. Fascial restrictions can lead to pain, restriction of motion, and a multitude of symptoms.

Myofascial release principles are safe and highly effective for everybody. I cannot more strongly recommend that you follow Nikki's advice. She has an amazing perspective with how to treat her patients.

– John F. Barnes PT

# IMPORTANT NOTE

The advice given in this book is very general and cannot take into account your particular physical or medical condition. As such, this book is meant to be practical and informative but is not intended to be a substitute for professional advice. It is not meant to replace any relationship that exists between you and your doctor, hospital specialist or other healthcare professional.

It is essential that you only follow any of the advice or exercises suggested in this book if you feel that you are able to do so safely. If you are unsure about any element, you should consult a health professional before commencing any new exercise. If you carry out any of the exercises included in this book, you are responsible for your own safety and should stop immediately if you feel any undue effects.

# INTRODUCTION

## Why I wrote this book

I decided that I wanted to be a physiotherapist when I spoke to one at a school careers evening, aged thirteen. Luckily, this teenage choice led me to a profession that has taken me around the world, fits around my family commitments, and fulfils me every day.

In 1993, I graduated from the Queen Elizabeth School of Physiotherapy in Birmingham, after three years of training. My first job was at the Luton and Dunstable Hospital, where I spent two years rotating through the specialties, gaining a broad base of knowledge and experience.

From the beginning, I didn't feel I was suited to working in a hospital outpatients' department. I didn't like only being allowed to treat the part of my patient's body that the doctor mentioned on the referral letter. However, I loved working on the wards, where I was free to treat my patients in my own way, especially in trauma and orthopaedics.

After eighteen months, I was given a fantastic opportunity: I swapped jobs with an Australian physiotherapist and went to live and work in Victoria for three months. That led to various locum positions in Melbourne, with a fair bit of travelling along the way!

On my return to the UK, following a honeymoon backpacking through India and Nepal, I did some more locum jobs. Then I settled at the Thurrock Community Trust in Essex, as a superintendent physiotherapist. This gave me wonderful experience in working within a great multidisciplinary team and managing community therapists.

In 2001 I left to look after my baby twin boys, who were joined by a baby sister three years later. As you can imagine, this took up all my time and energy for a few years! But when my daughter started playgroup in 2006, I decided to set up my own physiotherapy practice. That was when I remembered that I didn't enjoy outpatients.

So, I started researching some courses that I could take to update my skills, and that is how I came across myofascial release. This is a gentle hands-on treatment that works with your body to find and treat the cause of your symptoms.

After the first five minutes of my first myofascial release course, I felt that I had come home. It sounds corny, I know, but suddenly all my concerns about working with outpatients fell away.

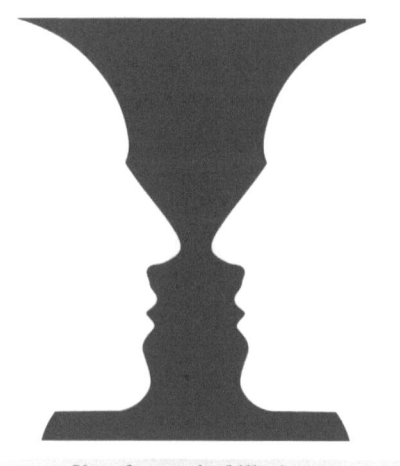

*Vase face optical illusion*

This is the illustration that had an immediate impact on me.
In all those years of treating people, I had been looking at the wrong picture! By learning how to observe and feel in the correct way, I felt that I was now able to work with my patients to change their symptoms.

I specialised in myofascial release straight away, and it has taken me on an amazing personal and professional journey that still continues today.

My initial myofascial release courses were in the UK, and I then trained in America with John Barnes, the physiotherapist who developed the technique. But, of course, learning is a continuous process and I still travel to the US to train with him whenever I can.

Since specialising in myofascial release, I have worked with thousands of patients who have had a huge variety of symptoms and conditions. The scope of this treatment continues to amaze and impress me.

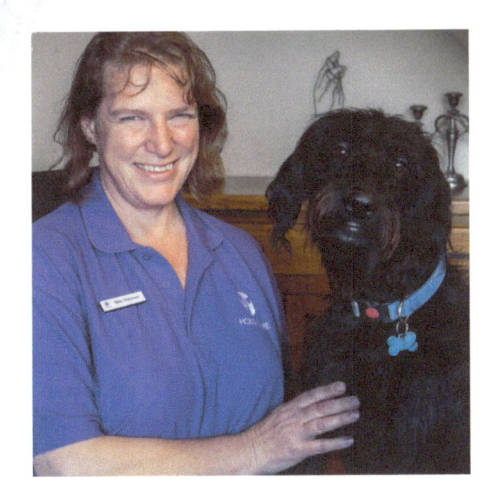

## How to use this book

This book is easy to pick up and browse, giving simple, practical, and common-sense tips on how to manage your pain. If you have a specific problem that you need help with, you can just turn straight to that section to find what you are looking for. You won't have to read it cover to cover, and there are plenty of photographs and illustrations to explain each point.

However, if you do enjoy reading a book from start to finish, there is a lot of information and explanation of how your body works and why you feel what you feel, relating to the latest research. This leads on to practical advice that is applicable to everyday life. If you would like to find out more details about the facts, there are references throughout the book for you to use.

## Is this you?

If you relate to any of these statements, this book could help you to find the answers:

- I am in constant pain or discomfort.
- My sleep is often disturbed by pain.
- I can't do the activities I want to because of my pain.
- I need daily medication to control my pain.
- I can't stand or walk for very long.
- I can't exercise as much as I would like to because of my symptoms.
- I am always conscious about my posture.
- I have to plan my days around my body.

- I usually manage my symptoms but sometimes a small event can make everything flare up.
- If I have a good day, I tend to overdo it, because I have to make the most of it.
- I can't keep up with friends of the same age as me.
- I have to take my own pillow if I go away.
- My body stiffens up overnight.
- I feel as though I am tied up in knots.
- Stretching helps, but I can't get far enough.
- I find it difficult to stand straight when I get up from sitting.
- It is very difficult for me to relax.
- I get very anxious and frustrated about my symptoms.
- I find myself waiting for my pain to return.
- I have been told it's all in my head.
- There is no point in having more treatment as I have tried everything.
- I have to ignore my body to get through the day.
- I have been told that my pelvis is out of alignment.
- I was given orthotics, but they didn't make any difference.
- My bite is out of line.
- I feel off balance.
- One of my legs feels longer than the other.
- I have tried lots of different treatments.
- I have been told that I can't be helped.
- My symptoms move around and change.
- My symptoms don't all fit into one diagnosis.
- My body is hypersensitive.

# CHAPTER 1

# YOUR FASCIA

## The ideal body and what can go wrong

The reality is that we are not made up of bones stacked up one on top of the other. Some of my patients with the most tension and the worst posture are those who were told as children to stand up straight and keep their shoulders back. Some were even made to walk round with a stick across the back of their shoulders! This has resulted in a spine that is ramrod straight and shoulders held in extreme tension. While their body is being held in this way, their whole system is put under so much pressure, they are unable to adapt to any stresses that come along.

Did you know that most people are walking around with a wonky pelvis?

Your pelvis is made up of two bones and the muscles attaching into those bones are the strongest in the body; those in your legs, back and stomach.

Postural Pelvic Malalignments

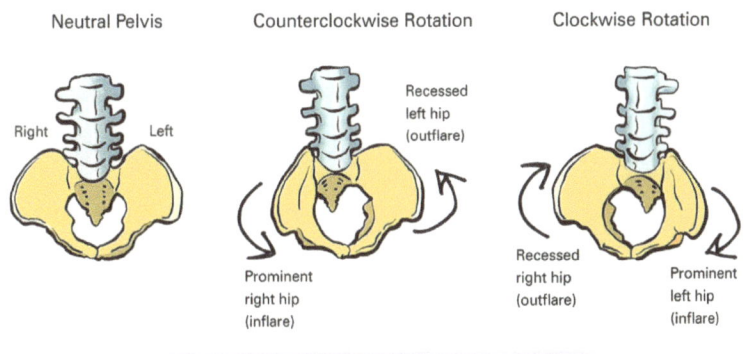

Neutral Pelvis — Right, Left

Counterclockwise Rotation — Recessed left hip (outflare); Prominent right hip (inflare)

Clockwise Rotation — Recessed right hip (outflare); Prominent left hip (inflare)

*Pelvic rotation*

Throughout your life, injuries and strains on those muscles cause them to tighten up. If they tighten up asymmetrically, they exert a rotational force on the bones of your pelvis; this causes the pelvic bones to gradually creep out of alignment. Because it happens slowly, the brain adapts to it, so most people are unaware that their pelvis is out of alignment. It can make you feel that you are off-balance and often people are told that one leg is longer than the other. It can also throw your shoulders and jaw out of position.

Your skeleton only has the structure that it has because of the soft tissue holding the bones in their relative positions. Without it, you would simply be a pile of bones. So, if your muscles are tight, your whole skeleton will be pulled out of position. This makes it extremely difficult to achieve a toned and balanced posture. Muscles can appear weak if they are tight or twisted.

Muscles in your body tend to work in pairs, often front to back – for example, your biceps muscles and your triceps muscles in your upper arm. In order for one muscle to work effectively (the agonist), its opposite muscle must be able to relax (the antagonist).

Muscles working in pairs

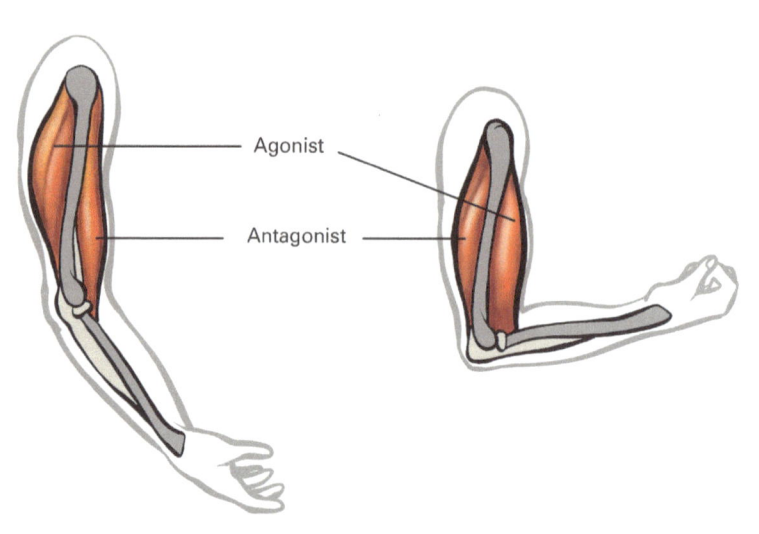

*Agonist/antagonist muscles*

Therefore, if you have tension that you can't let go of, the opposite muscle group will not be able to work correctly. This will have a big impact on your posture. A common example of this is when your shoulders are rounded or pulled forward. It is often seen with a head-forward posture too. Chapter 7 on page 79 has self-treatment techniques that can help if this is an issue for you.

## What is your fascia?

It used to be thought that the fascia was a white filmy covering that surrounded the organs and muscles, holding them in place. This has now proved to be incorrect, and I am very excited to be working as part of the fast-growing world of fascia therapy, which is being backed up by many new strands of research.

Your fascia, or connective tissue, is a three-dimensional network of microscopic hollow tubules that joins every one of your cells together. This web is continuous with a network of fibres within each cell that connects with the nucleus. So, there is no part of your body that is not connected to every other part via your connective tissue.

This continuity is nicely illustrated in this photo of half a lemon. You can see that the lemon is made up of different parts – the skin, pith, segments, and the pulps (containing the juice) – which have different functions. But at no point is there any separation between the parts. They make up a continuous system with differentiated areas.

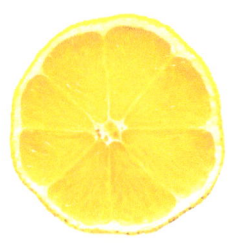

*Lemon – Photograph courtesy of @zcalvertl via Twenty20*

Your fascia is made up of:

- Collagen fibres within the tubules that give you strength and stability.
- Elastin fibres within the tubules to allow flexibility.
- The ground substance that sits between your cells and fibres. This gel-like substance is made up of water, hyaluronic

acid, and proteoglycans
It provides the correct environment for your cells to function properly and allows the fibres to move and change with the stresses and strains that are put on your body.[1]

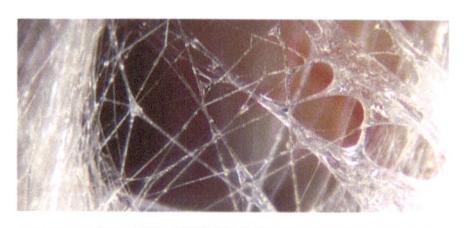

*An image of the fascial network, showing the interconnectedness of the fibres. Photograph courtesy of Dr. J.C. Guimberteau.*

In healthy conditions the fascial system is relaxed, providing strength, shape, flexibility, protection, and shock absorption, allowing you to move safely without restriction or pain. It is very strong, yet highly flexible and dynamic, adapting the position of its fibres depending on the stresses and strains put on it.[2]

If you had no restrictions within your fascial system, your body would have the ability to come back to its ideal position; even if it was put under strain by trauma or repetitive movements, it would be able to spring back once the strain was removed.

But the ground substance solidifies in response to trauma – for example, a sudden impact – or over time if there is constant irritation, such as a repetitive movement. This is a very similar reaction to corn flour – when you mix it with water to the right consistency, it becomes a non-Newtonian liquid. This means that it behaves like a liquid at times and a solid at other times. Custard and ketchup are other examples of things that react in this way.

When your ground substance solidifies, the cells can't function correctly, which may lead to disease and inflammation, and the fibres are unable to adapt to change, so they tighten up, leading to pain and tension. This in turn causes restrictions in other parts of the body, creating abnormal pressure. This crushing pressure affects the nerves and blood and lymphatic vessels, and further increases the tension in pain-sensitive structures. It also makes you more prone to injury. Symptoms such as pain, stiffness, tingling, and numbness may be due to this.

When you are moving, it is your fascia that enables you to sit and move in the way that you want, when you want, and to feel and respond to your surroundings.

## Biotensegrity

Architect and inventor Buckminster Fuller first talked about tensegrity in the 1970s, coining the term by combining the words *"tension"* and *"integrity."*

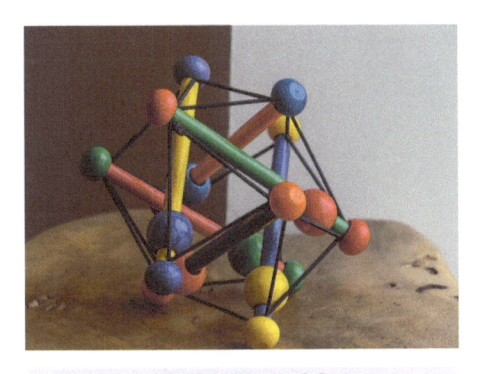

*Tensegrity model*

A tensegrity model is a structured system where the forces that compress it and those that put it under tension are balanced out. So, changing any part of the system will have an effect on all the other parts. As you can see in this photo, if you were to cut one of the elastics or break one of the sticks, the whole structure would collapse. But when they are all intact and working as they should do, then the model is very strong, but flexible. Then, if you imagine a knot in one of the elastics, pulling it shorter, you can see that the sticks it is attached to will also be pulled. This in turn will alter the position of the other ends of those sticks, and pull on the elastics at those ends, and so on.

When this system is seen in biological structures, including humans, it is called biotensegrity. Graham Scarr describes the human anatomy as a 'network of structures under tension and others that are compressed; parts that pull things together and others that keep them apart.'[3]

This system enables your body to adapt in a simple, efficient way to cope with forces that are potentially damaging. But once you add in scar tissue or other restrictions, they change that balance between tension and compression. Then, just like with the tensegrity model, the pull from the damaged part of your body will change the position and dynamics of every other part.

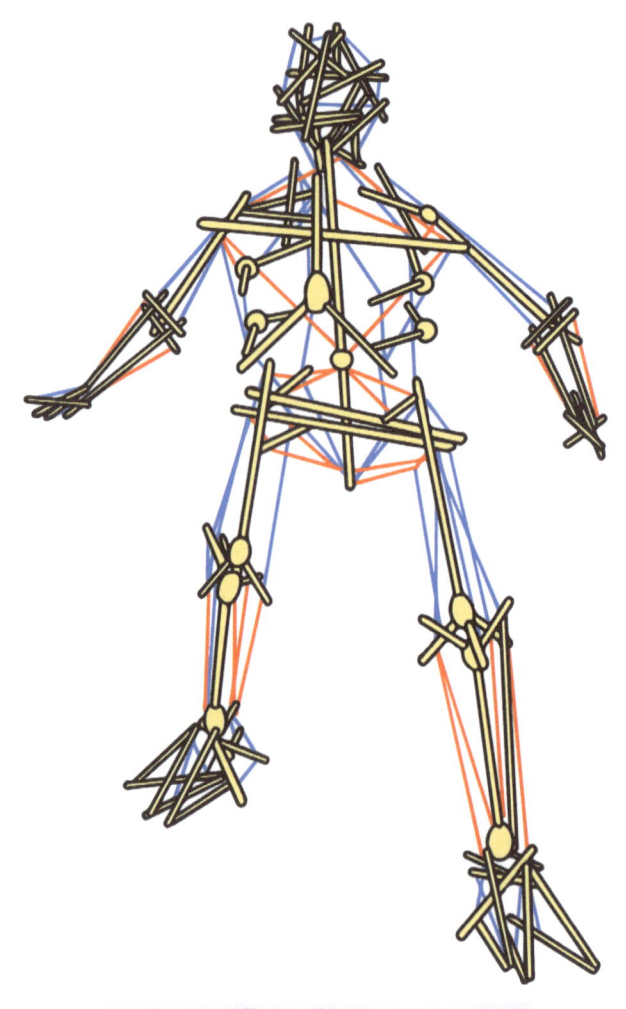

*Tensegrity man*

Biotensegrity is starting to explain how living systems are able to store energy for movement while maintaining stability. This property of your body is what allows you to move and change in response to the stresses and strains put onto you, without losing your shape and structure.

Traditional models of medicine tend to focus on your skeleton, describing the bones as the fundamental load-bearing structures into which all the muscles attach. Our understanding of biotensegrity tells us that actually your bones are merely the levers, and it is your fascial system that gives you your shape. This is such a different way of thinking about how our bodies are structured and how they work that the medical profession has been quite slow to take it up. But slowly, the research is spreading, and the profession is beginning to look at bodies from a different perspective, just like the vases in my introduction.

Dr. Jean-Claude Guimberteau is a French hand surgeon who has led the way in recording and researching the architecture of the myofascia. His images beautifully show the continuity of the fibres and how they are able to respond to changes in their environment and the forces acting on them. He describes how the system is 'mobile, can move quickly and interdependently, and is able to adapt its plasticity.'[4]

There are no straight lines in your body; all the different parts that work so brilliantly together to make the whole that becomes you are based on spiral shapes, fractals, and branches, which are found everywhere in nature.

The Romanesco cauliflower in this photo demonstrates this property beautifully.

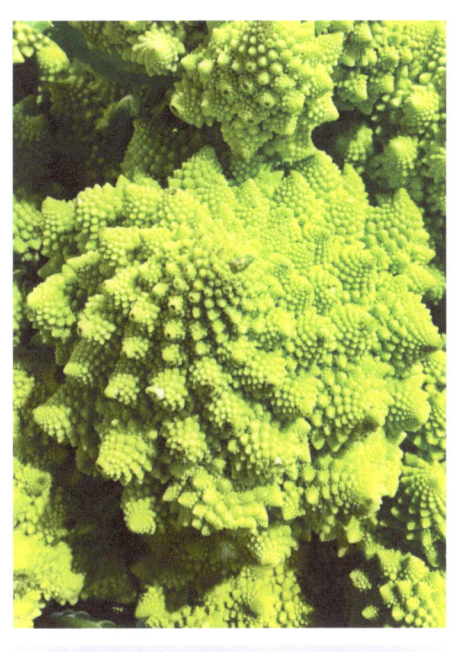

*Romanesco cauliflower – Photograph courtesy of @Ifusco via Twenty20*

We are very used to seeing these beautiful repeating patterns in nature, but the idea that we are also made up in the same way is very new to most of us. When you are aware of it, you can see bodies in a completely different light. The biotensegrity model explains that all your movements come from the interaction of repeated shapes within your body at all levels.

## References

1. L. Chaitow and J. DeLany. *"Clinical Application of Neuromuscular Techniques."* Vol. 1, The Upper Body. 2nd ed. Philadelphia, PA: Churchill Livingstone, 2008.

2. R. Schliep, T. W. Findley, L. Chaitow, and P. A. Huijing, eds. *"Fascia: The Tensional Network of the Human Body."* Philadelphia, PA: Churchill Livingstone, 2012.

3. G. Scarr. Biotensegrity: *"The Structural Basis of Life."* Pencaitland, Scotland: Handspring, 2014.

4. J.-C. Guimberteau. *"Architecture of Human Living Fascia."* Pencaitland, Scotland: Handspring, 2015.

# CHAPTER 2

# HOW YOUR BODY REACTS TO INJURY

*Please remember that the advice given in this chapter is general in nature and if you require individual advice, you should consult your own therapist.*

## Physical reaction

Your entire fascial network is continually responding to your environment, adapting to the stresses and strains that it is subjected to. This is its function: absorbing shock and flexing with the forces that are applied. But these changes should only be temporary to allow your system to survive the injury, and then your fascia should gradually come back to its normal, relaxed state.

In normal conditions your body should be able to fully relax when you are resting but be ready to instantly spring into action if you are in danger. This balance is managed by your autonomic nervous system, which regulates your body's functions without you needing to have conscious control of them. There are two parts of the autonomic nervous system, which between them balance the reactions of your internal organs to your environment.

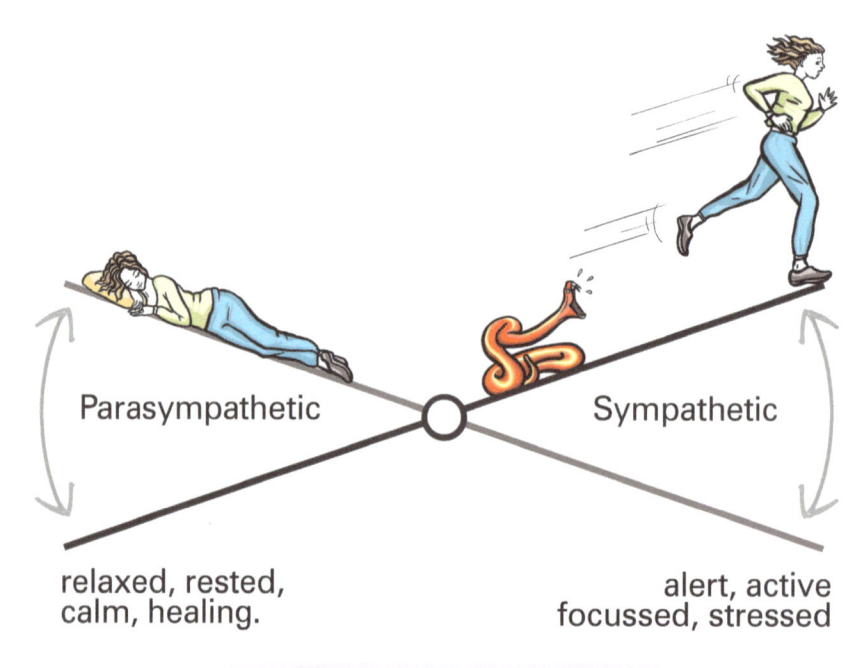

*The autonomic nervous system*

The sympathetic nervous system is stimulated when you are in danger (or perceived danger) and this is what produces the fight-or-flight response. Your adrenal glands release hormones, including adrenaline and cortisol, preparing your body for whatever it has to do to survive the dangerous situation. This has the effect of increasing your heart rate and blood pressure, expanding the air passages in your lungs, enlarging your pupils, and sending more blood to your muscles. This may save your life in an emergency, as you can find increased strength to defend yourself and improve your reaction times.

The parasympathetic nervous system has the role of conserving and restoring. It regulates your organs under normal conditions, and, after danger has passed, it slows your heart rate and decreases your blood pressure. It also stimulates your digestive system to allow energy from food to heal and build your tissues. That is why people very often hear their tummy rumbling during a relaxing treatment.

## Reactions to perceived danger or stress

The psoas muscles, also known as the fight-or flight muscles, are a pair of your core muscles and you have one on each side.
They run from the front of your hips, through your pelvis, and attach to the front of your lower spine. These muscles are responsible for a lot of people's back pain and stiffness.

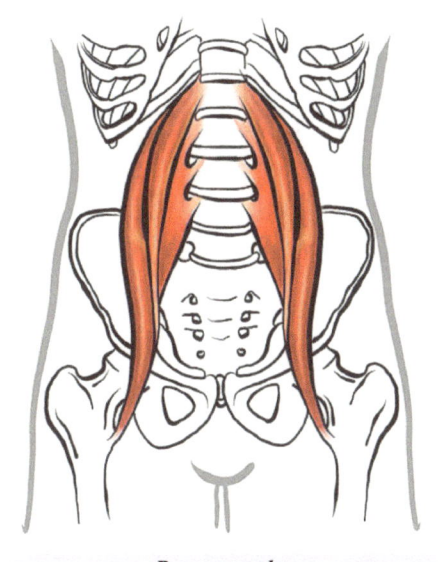

*Psoas muscles*

Their main action is to flex your hips, but they also help to stabilise the base of your spine. The psoas muscles are the only muscles that connect your trunk to the lower part of your body and pass from the front to the back of your body.

When you are stressed, in a dangerous situation, or have physical trauma, your sympathetic nervous system causes the psoas muscles to tighten. This protective response should only last for a couple of hours at the most, but for many people the tension is never released, and it becomes normal to them.[1]

The protective foetal position that anxiety throws your body into causes a flexed posture, where your upper body is tipped forward and your centre of gravity is further forward.

Another trauma response that is less recognized is the freeze or immobility response. This is a very primitive reaction, which is better known in the animal world. Think of a mouse that has been hunted by a cat. Even if it has not been badly injured, it will become immobile while the cat is still around. This survival instinct is to give it the best chance of escaping if the cat gets bored and becomes distracted by something more interesting. But if the poor mouse remains the focus of attention and the cat tosses it around and then eats it, the immobility response keeps it in what Peter Levine calls an 'altered state of consciousness,' where it will feel no pain or awareness of suffering.[2]

If an animal (especially a prey animal in the wild) survives the dangerous event or a potential threat, it does not just carry on as though nothing has happened. It will go through a period of intense shaking once the danger has passed, to burn off the excess energy that has been released. Once this has been completed, its system can return to normal, and it is unlikely to carry that trauma with it in the future. It will go through this cycle many times a day without long term ill effects, by simply following its body's natural reactions.

My dog has a shake after every time she pulls on the lead and her collar tightens. She is not in pain, but the tension that has come into her system needs releasing. How many times a day would your tension need to be released?

Owing to our ability to override this primitive reaction, our bodies retain the cell memory of the trauma, and we have to compensate for that as long as it remains. Over our lifetimes, each frozen memory is layered onto the previous traumas, until we feel that we are encased in concrete. Then the fibres of our fascial system are unable to move and change as they need to, our cells cannot function as they should, and we end up with pain and disease.

This is why you often see athletes with the same injury over and over again. The layers of compensation make it very difficult to fully recover from traumas, and the tension created by each new incident joins the old holding patterns in your body.

## Emotional response

Many of us live in a permanent state of fight or flight, possibly because of previous traumas, or the stresses of everyday modern life. If our system is already on high alert, it does not take much in the way of extra stress to tip us over the edge into full-blown panic or meltdown.

As explained in the previous sections, your system carries tissue and cell memory. This does not record only past physical traumas, but the associated emotions too. This is why some situations instantly catapult us back to old memories, feelings, or reactions.

For example, I once treated a patient with a very deep scar on the side of his thigh from a bad accident. As soon as I touched the scar, he began to sweat and to feel extremely nauseous and anxious. Then he told me that after the surgery to repair his bone, which was nearly 50 years previously, his bone had become infected, and he was extremely ill afterwards. Even though the infection and bone had healed many years ago, the trauma of that time was still held within the fascia of this scar tissue.

If you have suffered a trauma, your fascial system and subconscious mind will have recorded the position that you were in at that point. Your mind then associates that particular position with danger or pain, so it will try to avoid it as much as possible. Have you ever noticed that some movements have a funny kink in them, or that if you try to do a certain movement it doesn't feel safe, so you just don't do it?

As far as your mind is concerned, the danger that you are reacting to doesn't have to have happened. You know that feeling when you think that the lorry is going to hit your car? The shot of adrenaline that flies through your system at that moment when you think that you are going to get seriously hurt is as real as the adrenaline that is released when you are actually injured.

In this way, old injuries and traumas (physical or emotional) lead to compensations that can affect you every day of your life. So, it doesn't take much to shift your body from just about coping into spasm, pain, and inflammation. The thing that pushes you over your limit is often stress.

Stress has become the normal state for many of us, and over time it has an effect on the mind and body. Your brain interprets the tension as a sign of danger and keeps the sympathetic nervous system on high alert. This cycle of chronic stress can lead to pain, tightness, fatigue, and breathing and digestive problems. Your fight-or-flight response is only meant to be in place for a couple of hours or days at the most. However, a lot of people are living in a permanent state of fight or flight, which affects their physical and emotional health.

If your stress response continues, it stops being helpful and can damage your health, immunity, mood, and quality of life, adding to the feelings of stress and anxiety. Then it is quite easy to trigger an extreme reaction like a panic attack or hyperventilation. It may also result in phobias.

Consider the stress cycle shown in the illustration. Is this pattern familiar to you?

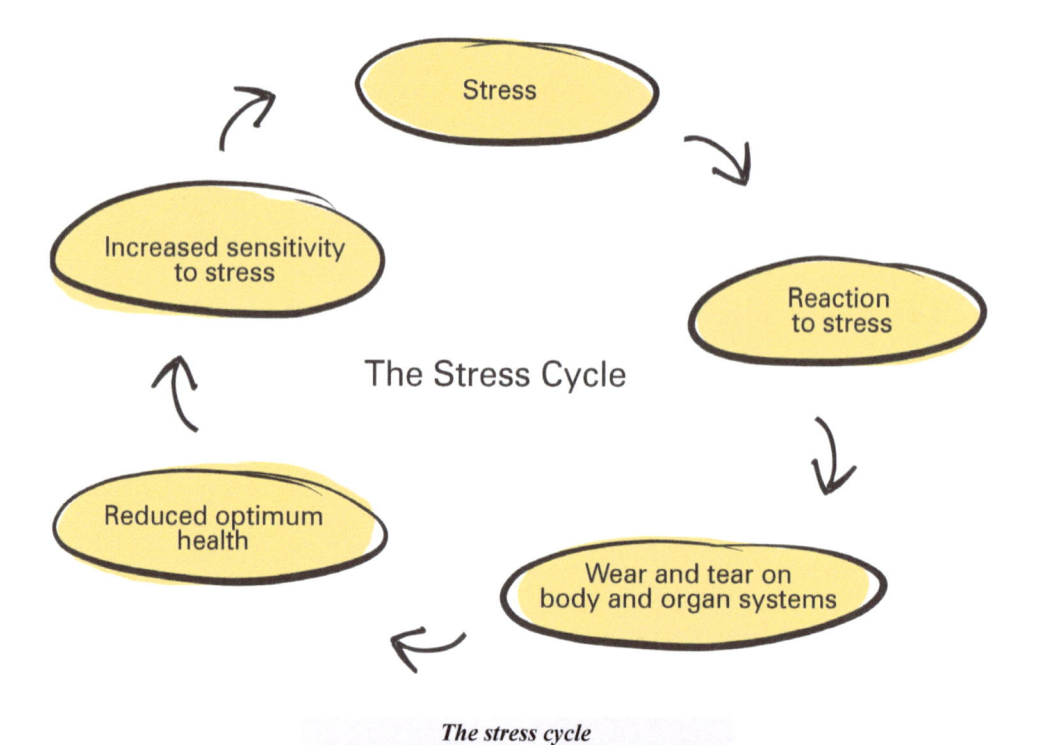

*The stress cycle*

This chain of events often leads to chronic pain and conditions such as fibromyalgia and chronic fatigue syndrome. It is the restrictions that are held in your fascial system that cause the reactions that lead to tension and the resulting physical and emotional illness.

### *How to help yourself:*

- Identify your stress triggers and try to change or manage them.
- Even if you can't alter the situation, changing your reaction to it can still help.
- Set aside regular relaxation time.
- Exercise regularly, even it is just going for a walk.
- Eat a healthy diet.
- Get plenty of sleep.
- Find a local yoga or tai chi class and use the moves yourself every day.
- Learn mindfulness or meditation as a way of managing your daily stress.
- Accept the things you can't change.

### *If you have a panic attack:*

A panic attack is when your body exaggerates its normal response to fear. They can be very frightening but cannot harm you physically or mentally. According to the No Panic website[3], common symptoms are:

- Breathing difficulties.
- Pains or tightness of the chest.
- Palpitations.
- Feeling unreal or not there.
- Dizziness.
- Trembling.
- Sweating.
- Feeling faint or loss of balance.
- A fear of not being in control.
- A feeling that you can't cope.
- A feeling of being trapped.
- A feeling of losing control.

If you feel that a panic attack is starting, there are a few things that you can do to reduce the feelings and calm things down:

- Breathe out slowly: your natural reaction to stress is often to keep trying to breathe in but forgetting to breathe out first, so you end up with a lungful of stale air.
- Check your posture: are you hunched over with your shoulders up around your ears? This position feeds

back to your brain that you are under stress, even if you are not.
- Don't fight or run away from your symptoms– they will not harm you and accepting them will help you to regain control faster.
- Remember that this is a normal reaction to stress and anxiety.
- If this is happening regularly, consider getting help from a trained professional who can help you to identify the reasons for your panic attacks and work with you to reduce your reactions.

More help with how to breathe properly can be found in chapter 5 on page 57.

## Falls

*A few statistics:*[4]

- 'A survey commissioned by Age UK has found that millions of older people are worried about falling over, with 4.3 million (36%) saying it topped their list of concerns.'
- 'Falls are the most common cause of injury related deaths in people over the age of 75 with over 5,000 older people dying as a result of a fall in 2017, a 70% increase on the numbers in 2010.'

Even relatively minor falls cause an impact and affect your whole body via your fascial system, but if there is no major injury, falls are often ignored. The effect of the impact might not be in the part of the body that you landed on. The transmission of forces through your body should allow the shock of the impact to be distributed and not focused in one place. But old fascial restrictions block the shock and cause it to get stuck within the fascial network. This causes new restrictions on top of the old ones, and new symptoms to develop over time that are separate from the immediate pain of the fall.

Your *"normal"* then becomes the tightness from old falls and injuries, as your brain gets used to it and stops telling you that there is a problem. Muscles can't work as effectively and can't be properly strengthened if they are tight and twisted.

So, the more impacts you have, the longer it will take to recover from injuries.

You may also tighten up and get a trauma response if you think you are going to fall, even if you don't. That is your protective mechanisms kicking in, as your sympathetic nervous system reacts to the perceived danger.
If you have had a near miss, try to give yourself time afterwards to let go of any tension that you are still holding on to.

## *How to help yourself after a fall:*

- Even if you don't think that you were hurt, give yourself time to feel your body before you get back up. Remember the impact will affect your whole body, not just the part that you landed on or that is hurting.
- If you have been winded, don't panic. That feeling of not being able to take a proper breath can feel quite scary and that anxious feeling then makes it even harder to breathe. The reason that you can't breathe easily is that the impact makes your diaphragm (the main muscle that you use for breathing) go into spasm. Sit in a crouched position and try to take slow, deep breaths, remembering to give yourself time to breathe out before you breathe in again. If things do not improve after about fifteen minutes, seek medical attention to check that you do not have more serious injuries.
- If you have any bruises or swelling, rest the area initially, and then try to keep it moving gently.
  You may find that applying a compression bandage helps to start with. For many years the advice was to use ice packs for injuries, but recently Dr. Gabe Mirkin, who originally gave that advice, has stated that using ice will delay healing and recovery. [5] This is because it narrows the blood vessels and limits the body's inflammatory response, which is essential for healing. He advises the use of ice packs for pain relief only in the first six hours after injury.

- Later in the day, try to gently stretch any tight areas, allowing your body to move as it needs to and not pushing into pain. For ideas on how to release specific areas, have a look at chapter 7 on page 79.
- If you had any trauma to your head, make sure that you follow the guidelines below.

## Concussion

Head injuries are starting to be taken seriously in many sports, such as horse riding, rugby and boxing. It is therefore important that everyone is aware of the symptoms to look out for following a blow to the head, and what to do about it. These guidelines are from the Headway website:[6]

If any of these signs are observed following a head injury, the person should be checked by a healthcare professional:

- Loss of consciousness.
- Increasing disorientation.
- New deafness in one or both ears.
- Problems understanding or speaking.
- Loss of balance or problems walking.
- Blurred or double vision.
- Any weakness in one or both arms or legs.
- Inability to be woken.
- Any vomiting.
- Bleeding from one or both ears.
- Clear fluid coming out of your ears or nose.
- Any fits (collapsing or passing out suddenly).
- Drowsiness when you would normally be wide awake.
- Severe headache not relieved by painkillers such as paracetamol.

Even if you do not suffer with any of these symptoms, a blow to your head is a significant trauma and should be taken into consideration if you go on to suffer any other symptoms in the future.

## References

1. J. A. Staugaard-Jones. *"The Vital Psoas Muscle."* Chichester, UK: Lotus, 2012.

2. P. Levine. Waking the Tiger: *"Healing the Trauma."* Berkeley, CA: North Atlantic Books, 1997.

3. Silvermarbles. *"Panic Attacks."* No Panic. https://nopanic.org.uk/how-to-overcome-panic-attacks/. Accessed 30th October 2022.

4. https://www.ageuk.org.uk/latest-press/articles/2019/may/falls-in-later-life-a-huge-concern-for-older-people/ Accessed 29th October 2022.

5. G. Mirkin. *"Why Ice Delays Recovery."* DrMirkin. 16 September 2015, last modified 2 May 2018. https://www.drmirkin.com/fitness/why-ice-delays-recovery.html

6. https://www.headway.org.uk/about-brain-injury/individuals/types-of-brain-injury/mild-head-injury-and-concussion/ Accessed 30th October 2022.

*Without awareness, there can be no change.*

John F. Barnes

# CHAPTER 3

# COMMON SYMPTOMS

## Pain

A British Medical Journal report found that chronic pain affects between one third and one half of the population of the UK, which is approximately 28 million adults.[1]

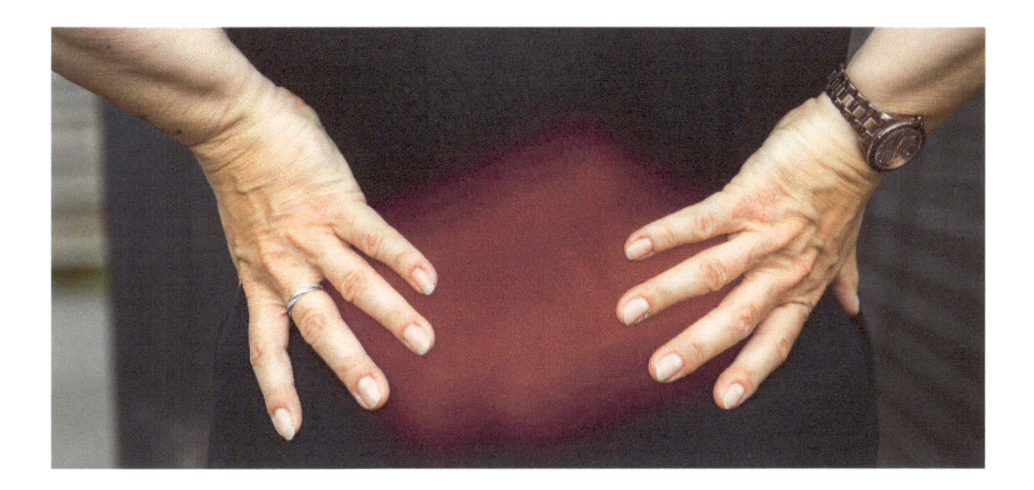

Pain is defined by the International Association for the Study of Pain as, 'an unpleasant sensory and emotional experience associated with actual or potential tissue damage, or described in terms of such damage.'[2]

This means that the mind and body cannot be separated, and everyone's perception of pain is different. The amount of pain felt doesn't only depend on how much damage has been sustained but will vary according to what has happened to you in the past.

The pain felt after an injury is a necessary, protective mechanism that makes you aware of the damage and ensures that you take action. It is a warning sign that needs to be acknowledged and responded to, not suppressed. But in some people, this mechanism becomes stuck, leading to chronic or long-term pain.

You feel pain when the nerve endings that are sitting within your tissues are stimulated. There are receptors to pick up lots of different sensations, and some of them are specialised to sense those that may be harmful, such as heat, pressure, or chemicals. They communicate those sensations via your spinal cord to your brain, which is when you feel them. When those sensations reach a critical level, you will feel them as pain.

If the nerve endings in a certain area are over-stimulated by constant irritation (such as pressure from the surrounding tissues or inflammation), even those that previously did not detect pain become pain sensitive. It has been estimated that fascial restrictions put up to 2,000 pounds per square inch of pressure on your nerve endings, which is the equivalent of a fully grown draught horse sitting on you![3] This is how chronic pain (lasting more than three months) develops.

When the pain pathways from your nerve endings are stimulated, the receptors in your brain interpret this as your tissues being damaged. Your brain sends pain-killing chemicals to the area and triggers an inflammatory response and the repair process. This is essential when you actually have hurt yourself, but it becomes a problem when the cycle is being continued not by a new injury, but by the continued pressure on the nerve endings from your fascial restrictions.

The pain cycle can become an issue if when an area is injured and then becomes swollen and inflamed, the resulting tightness and scar tissue further irritates it. The area never has a chance to settle, and the nerve endings keep telling your brain that there is damage, so the inflammation also becomes chronic, and the cycle continues.

## The Pain Cycle

- Repetitive use/injury/trauma
- Leading to inflammation
- Healing
- Building up adhesions and scar tissue
- Leading to tissue and nerve binding
- Resulting in pain and decreased range of motion

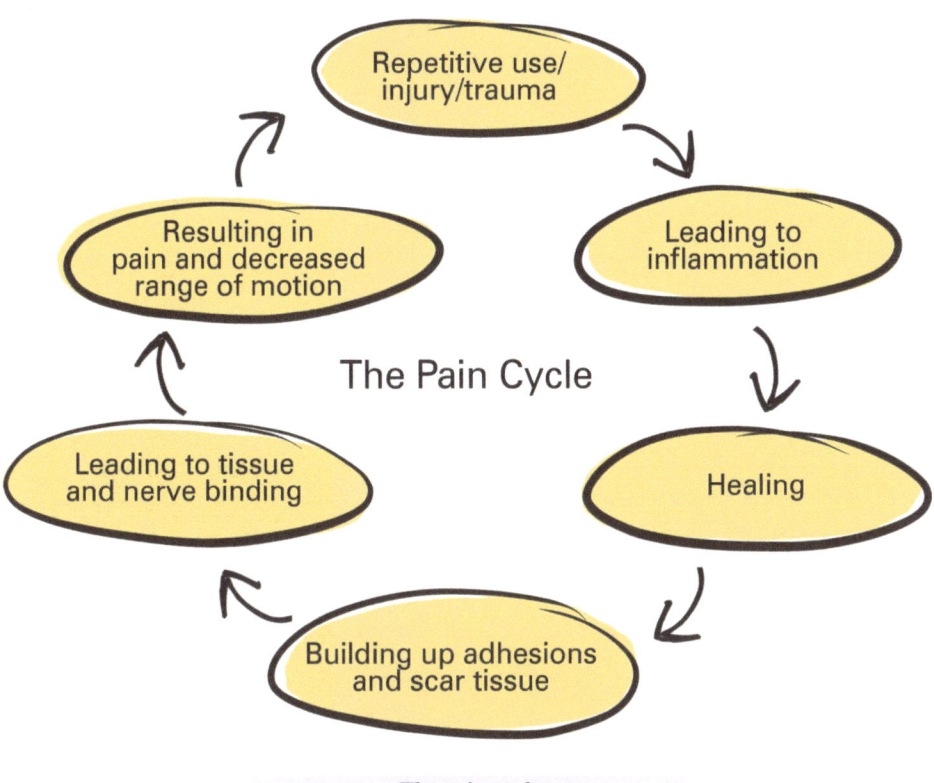

*The pain cycle*

Chronic pain affects all areas of life as it can lead to lack of sleep, fatigue, irritation, depression, and anxiety. People's relationships and jobs suffer, and previously enjoyable activities become difficult or even impossible.

Taking medication is the most common solution offered by doctors but remember that the cause of your pain may be in a completely different part of your body to where you are feeling the symptoms. Medical investigations to find out if there is any cause of your pain that needs immediate treatment is essential, but medication can mask what you are feeling and does not necessarily address the root cause.

There are some environmental conditions which will make things harder for everyone, even if you don't live with pain all the time. The weather is the main factor that can't be controlled, and prolonged spells of cold, wet weather will test even the most enthusiastic horse or dog owner. Being prepared by having the right clothing and equipment is the best way to get through those long winters.

Using heated seats or hot packs in your car will help your back to stay flexible, as at least you will start off by being warm. You can also get heated patches that stick to your clothes; these are particularly good for arthritic joints.

Do your joints let you know when damp rainy weather is coming without you needing to see the forecast? According to a study done by Harvard Medical School's Professor Robert Jamison, 67.9% of people surveyed felt the same. [4] He concluded that the increased pain may be due to a change in barometric pressure (atmospheric pressure), which normally pushes against the body from the outside. When the weather worsens, the barometric pressure falls, causing tissues in the body to expand and push on the nerve endings that signal pain.

## Tension

Why do you feel tight?

When your body is loose, relaxed and elastic, it can move and change with you. Over time it is very common to gradually feel tighter, but it isn't inevitable. My patients often tell me that they didn't realise that their tightness was anything that could be changed as they have had it for so long. They blame themselves for not exercising, living with stress, and getting older.

***There are several possible reasons for tension to build up in your tissues:***

- Dehydration: the fibres in your fascial system (as described in chapter 1 on page 7) need their environment to be fluid to allow them to move and adapt to the forces put on your body. If you are dehydrated, the fibres are less able to do this, and they become stuck and locked down. You will feel this as knots in your muscles and stiffness around your joints.

- Poor posture: if you spend most of your time in positions that put your body under strain, it will react by tensing up to protect itself. For example, looking down for long periods of time will result in tightness at the front of your neck, leading to tension in the back.
- Overusing muscles: as with poor posture, putting your muscles under pressure when they are fatiguing will cause the fibres in the area to tighten up to protect the muscles.
- Stress: one of the hormones produced by your body in response to stress stimulates your kidneys to resorb water from your system, which can lead to dehydration.
- Not stretching properly after exercise: muscles that have worked hard during exercise will naturally shorten as they cool down. If you do not create the conditions that allow them to open up again, that tension will remain.
- Pain or weakness in a different part of your body: this means that other areas of your body will need to work differently to compensate for the affected part not doing its job properly. The resulting imbalance causes tightness as muscles overwork.

As the pressure builds up in your muscles and they stiffen up, they gradually get thicker and shorter. This means that the blood flow isn't as good as it should be to help with healing, so you get more scarring, which makes the area even stiffer. Stretching opens up the layers of your muscles. It helps the blood flow and takes the pressure off the nerves, so pain and inflammation can be prevented or improved.

Remember that where you feel your symptoms is often different to where the cause of them is. Your tightness may be due to problems in another part of your body and is your body's way of compensating and trying to protect itself. So, there is no point in simply stretching the tight bit without also finding and treating the cause. If the tension is not released it can become a holding pattern in your body which has to then be compensated for, adding to the cycle of tension.

## Inflammation

Inflammation is a 'process by which your body's white blood cells and the things they make protect you from infection from outside invaders, such as bacteria and viruses.'[5]

Inflammation is an essential healing response that enables your body to respond to trauma and is a sign that your body is reacting in the correct way to the injury. There are different stages of the inflammatory response, and they need to be completed for full healing to occur.

The signs of inflammation are:

- Redness
- Swelling
- Tenderness
- Increased temperature
- Loss of function

*Stage 1:* this first, acute phase of healing lasts two to four days, when the aim is to start the healing process and to protect the area from further injury.
The blood supply to the injured area increases to bring chemicals and cells that assist with healing and remove damaged cells. This is when you will feel the most pain, warmth and swelling.

*Stage 2:* the second, sub-acute phase lasts up to six weeks and is the repair phase of healing. Scar tissue is formed but is still weak and vulnerable to further injury. Your pain and swelling should start to reduce in this stage.

*Stage 3:* the late, remodelling stage is between six weeks and three months after the initial injury. Your scar tissue begins to strengthen and become more organised in response to the loads that are put onto it. This is when it is important to move the injured area as normally as possible so that your body can heal in the correct way for the function required. Your range of movement and strength will improve during this stage.

Anything beyond three months is the chronic phase, which can continue for months after the injury.

The inflammatory healing process can be interrupted if the area is under strain. This may be coming from fascial restrictions in other areas or from overuse before the injury has had time to heal sufficiently. If this continues and the inflammation becomes chronic, it may lead to chronic pain too, as explained earlier in this chapter.

Inflammation does not only occur following an injury, though. As with the delay in healing, if an area is being constantly irritated by tension being transmitted through your fascial system, your tissues react as though they have been injured. Then, if the cause of the irritation continues, you will end up with chronic inflammation, which sometimes lasts for years.

This response is usually the root cause of conditions that seemingly appear for no apparent reason. For example, plantar fasciitis, tennis elbow, bursitis. They will be resistant to local treatment for as long as the irritation persists.

## References

1. A. Fayaz, P. Croft, R. M. Langford, L. J. Donaldson, and G. T. Jones. *"Prevalence of Chronic Pain in the UK: A Systematic Review and Meta-analysis of Population Studies."* BMJ Open 6, no. 6 (2016): e010364. doi:10.1136/bmjopen-2015-010364.

2. H. Merskey and N. Bogduk. *"Pain Terms: A Current List with Definitions and Notes on Usage."* Part 3 in Classification of Chronic Pain, 2nd ed., International Association for the Study of Pain (IASP) Task Force on Taxonomy. Seattle: IASP, 1994.

3. K. Kayate. 1961. *"The Strength for Tension and Bursting of Human Fasciae."* Journal of the Kyoto Prefectural Medical University 1969 (1961): 484–88.

4. R. N. Jamison, K. O. Anderson, and M. A. Slater. *"Weather Changes and Pain: Perceived Influence of Local Climate on Pain Complaint in Chronic Pain Patients."* Pain 61, no. 2 (1995): 309–15.

5. https://www.webmd.com/arthritis/about-inflammation Accessed 30th October 2022.

*What is a more healthy, positive way to believe and act now?*

John F. Barnes

# CHAPTER 4

# COMMON CONDITIONS

The conditions listed here are just some of the more common problems experienced by people. Some people are in constant pain in multiple areas and others might only ever have one problem.

Whatever you are feeling, please note that the advice given in this chapter is only a guide and can never replace medical assessment and treatment if that is what is required. If you are unsure, please do see your doctor or body worker. Remember that everybody has their own medical history, which builds up to give the pattern of symptoms over time. You could take ten people with identical symptoms and the cause and treatment would be different for each person. Because of this, the advice given here is very general, and it is essential to follow your own body and to trust what you feel.

## Auto-immune disorders

There are many conditions which are classified as auto-immune disorders, each with their own characteristics. They affect everybody differently. There are some common symptoms that a lot of people report and if you are able to manage these, it can be easier to cope with the underlying condition.

- Fatigue
- Joint pain and swelling
- Achy muscles

As well as making sure that you are well hydrated and trying to work with your body (see chapter 5 on page 57), treating yourself using the myofascial release principles can be very helpful. Which techniques you need, and when, will vary according to how you are feeling. Many of my patients who have these types of conditions find it difficult to feel what their body is telling them, as they are so used to pushing those feelings to the back of their mind.

Chapter 7 has a lot of techniques that you can use to treat different areas of your body. I would encourage you to try just one to start with, get used to the feeling of how your symptoms respond, and then add in other techniques as you need.

## Back pain

According to NICE, 'up to 60% of the adult population can expect to have low back pain at some time in their life.'[1]

Back pain can occur as a result of several different pathologies, and some people will have more than one problem contributing to their pattern of pain. These can include damage to muscles, tendons, ligaments, discs, and vertebrae. Having said that, most back pain is not related to anything serious, and by keeping moving, avoiding aggravating tasks, doing gentle exercise and stretches, it should be possible to control it.

An article was published in the Lancet[2] which examined the research into low back pain assessment and treatment. The conclusion was that there was very little evidence for most of the invasive investigations, X-rays, scans, injections and surgeries. They did show that some manual therapy was helpful, together with a graded exercise programme.

However, there are some 'red flag' symptoms which may indicate a more serious problem and if you are experiencing any of these, it is very important to seek medical attention so that you can be checked and treated if necessary, especially if they come on following trauma such as a fall. The symptoms to look out for are:

- Numbness or pins and needles between your legs, in the area which would be in contact with a saddle.
- Inability to pass urine.
- Urinary or bowel incontinence.
- Leg weakness.
- Extreme pain in both or one of your legs.

As discussed in chapter 3 on page 27, your psoas muscles are very important in stabilising your lower back. As they are attached directly into your spine, they cause pain and tension in your back when they tighten up. Even if the original cause of your pain is from something else, the psoas muscles will tend to join in, making your symptoms worse. It is always worth keeping the psoas released as well as treating whatever else is going on – see chapter 7 on page 79.

Intervertebral discs are the soft, gel-filled cushions that sit between each vertebra in your spine. They act as shock absorbers, while allowing safe movement of your spine. Spinal scans often report degenerative changes of the discs or wear and tear. This is a natural change as you age, and the water content of the discs reduces from the 80% that you are born with.

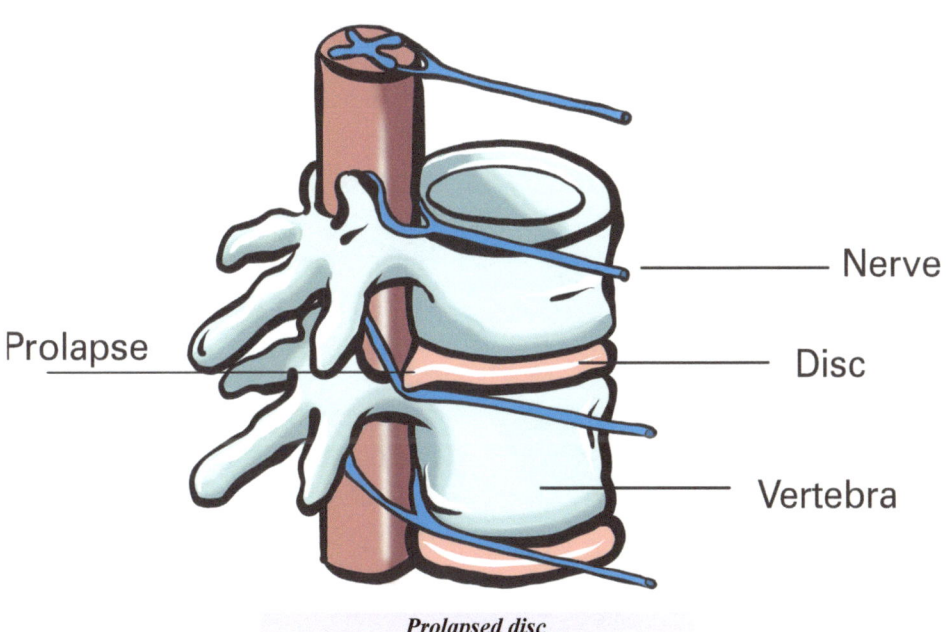

## Prolapsed Disc

*Prolapsed disc*

If a disc is compressed too much on one side, either by trauma or muscle tension, the gel is forced out to the other side (imagine what would happen if you filled a balloon with water and then squeezed it on one side). This pushes the disc out of its normal position and into the space occupied by the nerves; a slipped disc, resulting in very painful conditions such as sciatica and nerve pain down your legs. When seeking treatment for disc problems, it is important to remember that even though your pain may be on one side, the cause is probably on the other side. Relieve the compression and the disc will have space to come back into its rightful position, as long as it has not completely ruptured or displaced too much.

For ways to treat your back pain and tension, please look at chapter 7 on page 79.

## Bursitis

This is inflammation of the bursae, small fluid-filled sacs that cushion your joints. Bursitis can come on very quickly, causing pain, swelling, heat and redness in the area. Treatment is rest, ice, and gentle movement, remembering that the cause of the inflammation may be linked to problems elsewhere in your body – see chapter 3 on page 27.
If the symptoms last longer than a week, you should see medical attention. Hands-on treatment such as myofascial release can also be very beneficial.

## Fibromyalgia

Fibromyalgia is a chronic condition that causes widespread pain and fatigue all over the body. Sufferers often also report muscle stiffness and increased sensitivity. As this condition presents differently in each person and does not have a definitive diagnostic test at the moment, diagnosis is dependent on your doctor being aware of the condition and its implications.

Dr Ginevra Liptan is an American doctor who also has fibromyalgia, and she now specialises in treating patients with fibromyalgia and researching the condition. Her excellent book, The FibroManual, has a lot of information and if you are interested in finding out more,

I would recommend reading this and following her on social media as she regularly publishes updates on the latest research.

Although some fibromyalgia sufferers have to stop exercising altogether for at least a period of time, there are many who find that exercise is beneficial to their general well-being. This is a condition that is worsened by stress, so finding a low impact, enjoyable form of exercise that releases endorphins and helps to strengthen your core muscles is invaluable.

The advice in chapter 5 on page 57 is very helpful for managing the symptoms of fibromyalgia, especially the section on listening to your body.

Dr Liptan's research has found that people with fibromyalgia showed significant long-term benefits from myofascial release treatment.[3] Chapter 8 on page 111 has all the details on this treatment.

For ways to treat yourself, please look at chapter 7.

## Frozen shoulder

The symptoms of frozen shoulder are typically pain and stiffness in the shoulder joint. This can come on very quickly and without appropriate treatment it may last for months or even years. Sufferers struggle to use the affected arm for day-to-day activities and the pain may spread to the surrounding areas.

Like many inflammatory conditions, frozen shoulder often develops in response to restrictions elsewhere in the body. For example, if your pelvis is out of alignment (as discussed in chapter 1 on page 7) or you have scar tissue from old injuries or operations, your body needs to compensate. So, as well as trying to reduce the pain and stiffness, it is important to identify the cause of your frozen shoulder and treat that too. This is likely to need input from a bodyworker, but there are things that you can do to help yourself – see chapter 7 on page 79 for some self-treatment techniques.

## Hypermobility

People with hypermobility syndrome have the ability to move their joints beyond the normal range, eg, being able to bend their thumbs back on themselves. It is sometimes known as being double jointed. This trait is often passed down through families and there are different grades of severity.

Some families are identified as having a particular syndrome such as Ehlers-Danlos Syndrome (EDS), but many people do not realise they are hypermobile until they have a problem. But you can be hypermobile without having a serious condition. If you think that you may be hypermobile and are concerned about it, speak to your doctor, who will be able to run some tests and advise you on any treatment that you may need.

The hypermobility is caused by faulty collagen in your connective tissue fibres, which leads to looseness in structures throughout your body, such as ligaments and skin. The pain around joints, which is a typical symptom, is caused by recurrent soft tissue damage from repeated over stretching.

Core strengthening and joint stabilising exercises are the key to exercising safely if you are hypermobile. I am not going to give any specific exercises or releases here, as there are too many variables in the condition and therefore you need to be assessed in person by someone who is qualified to advise you. This may be a therapist with training in exercise prescription or someone such as a Pilates or yoga instructor who has experience in working with hypermobile people.

The releases that are shown in other sections of this book are very general and would normally be safe to do, even with hypermobility. However, I would strongly encourage you to seek individual advice, perhaps even showing your therapist or exercise instructor this book, before you start anything new.

## Incontinence

'It is estimated that around 7 million people in the UK have urinary incontinence (5-10% of the population).'[4]

Your pelvic floor is a sling of muscles that attaches to the bottom of your pelvis, supporting your pelvic organs and giving you control over your bladder and bowels. It is as important for men as for women, but often it is only mentioned or thought about after childbirth.

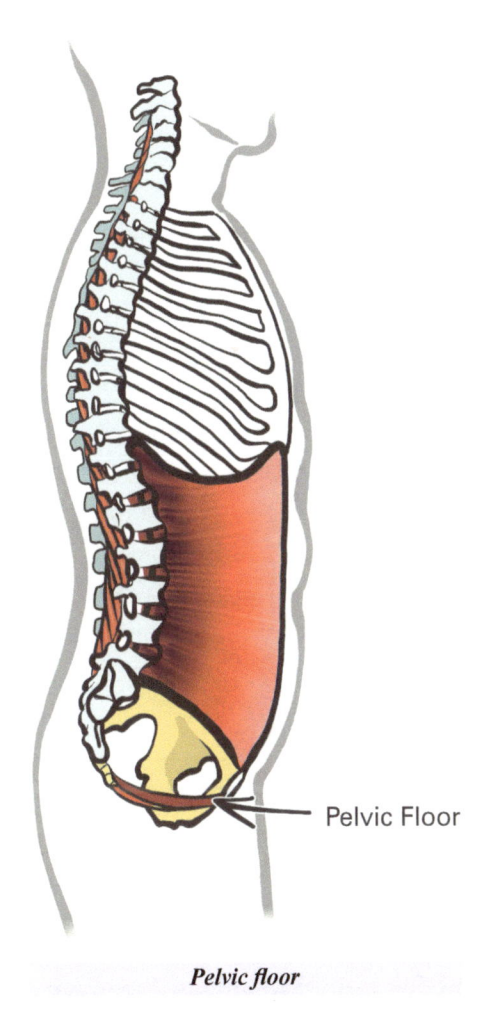

*Pelvic floor*

There are two main types of urinary incontinence: stress or urge, with some people suffering from both. The causes and treatment are the same for each type in most cases and men can be affected as well as women.

Stress incontinence is when the pelvic floor is unable to prevent urine from leaking when put under pressure. This may be when you cough, sneeze, or exercise.

Urge incontinence is the inability to stop urine flow when your bladder feels that it is full, sometimes called an overactive bladder. It is why some people will always go to the bathroom 'just in case' and will normally be very aware of when the next opportunity to go will be.

Urinary incontinence is normally blamed on a weak pelvic floor and sufferers are given exercises to strengthen it. This approach would be effective if that was the only reason – but remember that your pelvic floor is connected to the rest of your body, and it doesn't work in isolation. If you have a history that includes back pain, pelvic rotation, childbirth, surgery, or trauma (particularly in the abdominal or pelvic area) or pelvic organ prolapse, it is highly likely that they are contributing to the weakness.

Finding and treating the cause will be much more successful than doing exercises alone to try and overcome the problem. Once your pelvic floor is no longer tight and twisted because of strain from other areas of your body, the exercises will be much more effective.

**What to do about it:**

*Tell your doctor.* So many people are embarrassed by this problem that they don't talk about it to their doctor or even friends and family. This has created a taboo which perpetuates the problem. In the first instance it is important for your doctor to rule out any conditions that may need medical intervention. Generally, the sooner problems are investigated and treated, the quicker and more successful the treatment.

There is world-wide controversy at the moment surrounding the use of vaginal mesh implants to treat incontinence.

There are many women who have reported ill-effects from the plastic polypropylene that is used and as I write there are lawsuits in progress. This is a rapidly changing area as the investigations progress, so I would advise you to look into the most recent developments for yourself if you are considering this operation.

*Get treatment.* Find a therapist who is qualified in treating incontinence by looking at your whole body and finding the cause. They will then be able to advise you on when and how to do the pelvic floor exercises. Ideally, see someone who is qualified in assessing and treating your pelvic alignment; if the bones of your pelvis that the pelvic floor muscles are attached to are rotated, then it follows that your pelvic floor will also be twisted. For more information about your pelvic alignment, please see chapter 1 on page 7.

*Pelvic floor exercises.* Most women who have had children will have heard of Kegel exercises, but they apply to men too. These pelvic floor exercises were devised by Dr Arnold Kegel, an American gynaecologist in the 1940s.

## Pelvic Floor Muscle Contraction

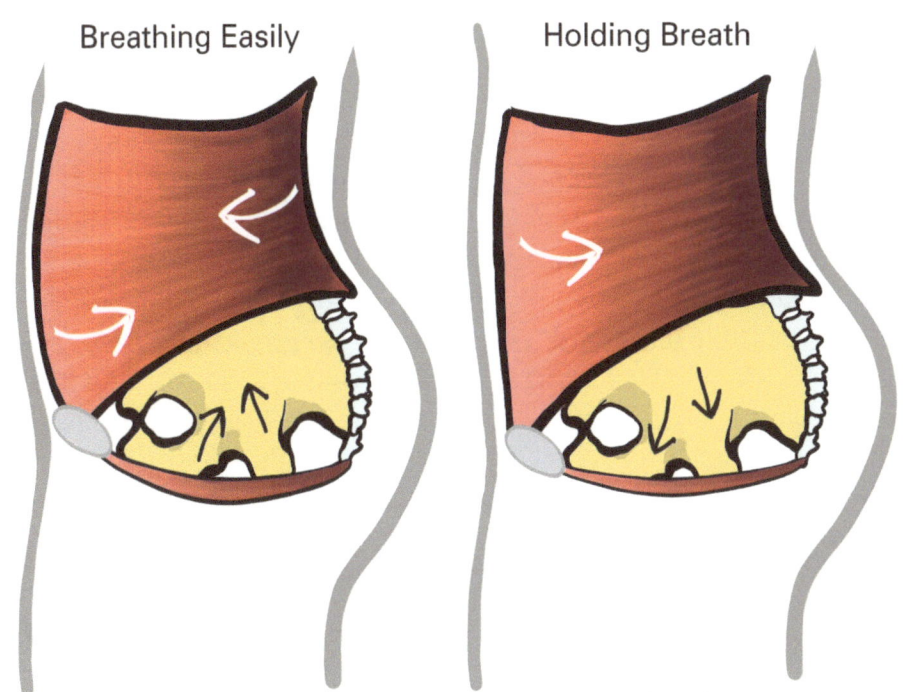

**Breathing Easily**

**Holding Breath**

Normal action
- The pelvic floor lifts.
- The deep abdominals pull in.
- Breathing stays the same.

Abnormal action
- Holding your breath pulls your belly button in towards your spine.
- This causes pressure down onto the pelvic floor.

*Pelvic floor muscle contraction*

Begin with an empty bladder and slowly contract your pelvic floor from the back to the front of your body, as if you are trying to stop yourself from passing urine. Then hold the contraction for a count of ten (you might need to build up to being able to maintain the contraction for that long) and slowly release the muscles until they are fully relaxed. Keep your breathing slow and gentle so that you do not hold your breath. Do not perform this exercise while you are passing urine, as it can lead to incomplete bladder emptying and an increased risk of urinary infection.

*Keep drinking.* Although it may seem counter-intuitive, it is very important to drink plenty of water to keep your bladder healthy. Limiting your fluid intake will increase the risk of infection and of bladder irritability. Sipping water throughout the day is a better way of keeping your body hydrated than gulping down lots in one go and is less likely to put a strain on your bladder if it is weak.

## Joint pain and stiffness

### Hand and wrist pain and stiffness

Common reasons for hand and wrist problems are arthritis, tendonitis, carpal tunnel syndrome, and fractures or dislocations to the fingers.

Whatever the cause, pain and stiffness in your hands affects most activities. There are simple changes that you can make that will help your hands to cope with the jobs you need them to do:

- Keep them warm and dry. Wearing a good pair of thermal gloves can make a huge difference to how your hands react to winter weather. This does sound really obvious, but I have seen people only think about putting on gloves once their fingers have gone numb and the joints are stiff. Prevention is much less painful! Disposable heat pads for gloves are great.

- Keep releasing them. As soon as you become aware of your fingers and hands tightening up, pause what you are doing, wriggle your fingers, circle your wrists, and stretch your hand gently open. See chapter 7 on page 79 for specific techniques.

### Elbow pain and stiffness

Elbow pain is most commonly due to tendonitis. Tendons are the strong bands that connect muscle to bone and 'itis' means inflammation. Tendonitis can occur anywhere in your body in response to ongoing tension and irritation. If it is the outer edge of your elbow that is sore, it is known as tennis elbow, and pain on the inner edge is called golfer's elbow.

Arthritis, as described earlier in this chapter, is often secondary to an old injury such as a fracture or dislocation, especially if surgery was needed at the time. Elbow injuries can be very problematic to heal, and people can be left with stiffness for the rest of their life.

If a patient tells me about trauma to their elbow in the past, I have come to expect that they will not be able to straighten it fully and to be a bit stiff and sore at the end of trying to bend it. Most of the time they have come to see me about a completely different part of their body as they just live with the pain and inconvenience of their old injury.

Get your neck and back checked. Most of the patients that I see with elbow pain have had a lot of different treatments and interventions, all to the elbow, and mostly with only temporary benefit. That is because some of the muscles attaching into your elbow link up to your shoulder.

Tension in your back and neck is very easily transferred into your shoulders and down your arms, irritating the tendons in your elbows and causing inflammation.

## Shoulder pain and stiffness

Shoulder problems typically present as pain and stiffness in and around the joint and are given different labels depending on the exact nature of the symptoms. In my experience, shoulder symptoms are normally connected to other areas of your body, even if there has been direct trauma to the shoulder joint. Your body should be able to heal injuries and inflammation, so if you are left with a chronic problem, the reason for it should be looked for elsewhere in your body.
For example, your pelvis might be out of alignment, or you may have scar tissue holding on to surrounding tissues.

If you have persistent shoulder symptoms, finding a therapist who specialises in a treatment like myofascial release can help to find and treat the cause.

## Knee pain and stiffness

The knee joint is very complex and is prone to injury and inflammation. Some common problems are arthritis, tendonitis, bursitis, ligament injuries, patella (kneecap) problems, and torn cartilage. Your knees often suffer from the strain put on them if your pelvis is out of alignment, if the muscles around your hips are tight, or if you are overweight.

The problem with most knee conditions is that because it is difficult to avoid the painful positions or movements, your body very quickly starts to compensate. Your knee joint relies a lot on your quadriceps (thigh muscles) to support it, but this group of muscles will weaken relatively quickly if they are not used properly. You will know if this is happening to you if your thigh tires quickly and your knee gives way suddenly.

Quadriceps muscle strengthening exercises should be taught face to face, as the person teaching you needs to check that you are doing the exercises correctly. If your knees ever give way or lock, see your doctor for tests and a referral to a therapist that is qualified to assess and treat you.

## Hip pain and stiffness

Your hips are particularly susceptible to inflammation and tightness, as they are directly articulating with your pelvis. As you will realise by now, if your pelvis has rotated and fixed in that position, your whole body has to compensate. But this is especially true of your hip joints and the soft tissue around them. Common hip problems include arthritis, bursitis, and tendonitis.

The tendonitis occurs because all the muscles in the area come under a lot of strain when the bones into which they are attaching are in the wrong position. The muscles which mainly affect your hips are your quadriceps (at the front of your thighs), hamstrings (at the back of your thighs), ilio-tibial band (IT band running down the outside of your thighs) and pelvic floor.

Finding a therapist who can check your pelvic alignment and balance the area is key to resolving a lot of hip issues.

## Joint replacements

Joint replacement surgery is most commonly carried out when joints become very stiff and painful due to arthritis. They are also sometimes performed following trauma, if the joint is unlikely to heal properly. Although most of these operations are seen as routine now, the recovery often involves some hard work to ensure that the new joint stays mobile, and the surrounding muscles are strong enough to support it.

Having treatment pre – and post-op can be very beneficial to prepare your body for the surgery and to speed recovery afterwards. Treating yourself around the new joint is also very important to reduce the effect of scar tissue on the surrounding area, maintain the circulation, reduce swelling, and control pain. The treatment will depend on which joint has been replaced and the specific instructions from the surgeon, but as long as it does not increase the pain, you can gently place your hands in the area of the joint to help the healing – as described in chapter 7 on page 79.

## Long Covid

Long Covid is thought to have affected over two million people in the UK. According to the NHS, it is defined as when symptoms last more than 12 weeks after getting Covid-19 and those symptoms cannot be explained by any other condition.[5]

Over 200 different symptoms have been reported and these may change over time. Recovery is very individual, but if you are experiencing new or concerning symptoms, it is important to seek medical advice and support.

The main ongoing issues tend to be breathlessness, pain, and fatigue. But many systems of the body may be affected: respiratory, cardiovascular, digestive, neurological and psychological.

### *Pace yourself*

Learning to listen to your body and pace yourself can be fundamental in helping yourself as you recover. Many people are used to ignoring what their body is telling them and pushing through their symptoms in order to continue with their lives as before. This can work if your

symptoms aren't too severe or if you only ignore them once. But continuing to ignore your body can actually increase symptoms and delay recovery. So, try to work with your body instead of against it.
For example, sitting to do some tasks that you would normally stand for, or taking a break halfway through a job.

### *Treatment for Long Covid*

Physiotherapy for Long Covid can help you to manage your symptoms. Myofascial release treatment can be beneficial and there are also specialist clinics that your GP may be able to refer you to.

The advice about breathing and pacing yourself in chapter 5 on page 57 should be helpful.

## Mental health conditions

The mind-body connection is now widely accepted as fact, and there is a growing body of evidence that demonstrates that 'the hormones and neurotransmitters associated with emotion can also have physical effects.'[6]

I regularly see examples of this in my patients; chronic pain leading to symptoms of depression, anxiety causing muscle tension and pain, and past traumas manifesting as inflammation. These are not direct cause and effect results, but more due to your body trying to compensate for ongoing stresses.

People living with conditions such as depression, anxiety and PTSD often also experience other symptoms like tension and pain. The self-treatment techniques in chapter 7 on page 79 are very helpful for this.

Speaking to your doctor about your symptoms is a good starting point, but there are many different therapies and organisations that can also help you. There is a list of some contacts in the UK for you at the end of this chapter. The most important thing is to ask for help and keep looking for solutions.

## Neck pain

Like back pain, your neck can be affected by the muscles, tendons, joints and ligaments in the area and the pain will be made worse if you are doing anything that puts strain on it.

If you have had any trauma to your head or neck and then you experience any of the following symptoms, it is important to get checked by a medical professional:

- Extreme pain in your neck or arms.
- Dizziness.
- Bad headache.
- Weakness in one or both arms.
- Urinary or bowel incontinence.
- Difficulty controlling your legs when walking.

Often pain that is felt at the back of your neck is due to tension in the muscles at the front – also linked to poor posture. As your head is relatively heavy and being upright against gravity requires you to be balanced, the muscles in your neck and upper back will tend to tense up to support your head and protect your neck.

The more you push your body while you have neck pain, the greater the protective response. This will result in tension being transmitted into your shoulders and down your arms.

This is when your shoulders are held up towards your ears, many times without you realising until you spot yourself in a mirror or someone else points it out to you. Holding your shoulders in this way may be associated with stress or it may simply have become a habit that feels normal.

When you are feeling stressed, your shoulders tend to creep up, which increases the tension in your muscles, causing pain, increasing stress, and so on until it becomes a vicious circle. The trouble is, once this becomes your normal position, your brain gets desensitised to it, and it is harder to pick up when it is happening.

Some people live their lives with their shoulders up round their ears, and others get the shoulder creep when they do certain things. If you are cold, nervous or stressed, it is more likely to happen.

The main muscle causing your shoulders to rise in this way is called the upper trapezius. This muscle is the upper part of the larger trapezius muscle and is the hard knotted area between your neck and the top of your shoulder.

For ways to treat your neck pain and tension, please look at chapter 7 on page 79.

## Neurological conditions

While myofascial release treatment does not replace neuro physio rehabilitation, it is an excellent adjunct to it in the early stages of stroke recovery. In the later stages, when rehabilitation may have slowed, myofascial release can be very beneficial in improving function. This is because many patients have symptoms after a stroke such as pain and tension, which are not directly related to the original brain injury but are due to compensation for the stroke. We have found that working with these patients to release the compensatory pain and tension can often result in better movement and mobility. As well as the hands-on treatment and advising on self-treatment techniques, we can show carers how to help manage their patients' symptoms every day at home.

This approach is also helpful in conditions such as Parkinson's disease and multiple sclerosis.

## Osteoarthritis

Osteoarthritis is sometimes known as wear and tear or degeneration of a joint. It can occur in any joint of the body and is a result of either abnormal use of a normal joint or normal use of an abnormal joint. In other words, you are much more likely to develop osteoarthritis if you were born with congenital abnormalities, if you have ever injured the joint, or if the joint is used over and over again in the same way.

The bony ends that come together to form the joint are covered by a thin layer of cartilage that protects them and produces joint fluid for lubrication. As the joint begins to degenerate, this layer is gradually worn away so there is less lubrication and more friction between the bone ends. Severe arthritis is when there is very little cartilage left and the bone ends themselves start to wear.

Osteophytes are extra areas of bone that the body lays down to try and repair the damage done by the arthritis. They are normally located on the outside of joints and look like nodules. They can cause a lot of pain as they push on nerves in the area that they grow in and lead to inflammation around them.

Typical symptoms are stiffness if you haven't moved for a while, especially first thing in the morning, and pain. Both symptoms will get worse if you do too much. You can also get swelling around the affected joint and extra bone that is laid down by the body as it tries to correct the damage.

As with other painful conditions, it is the tension around the joint that causes most of the problems. This is because your other muscles need to work differently to maintain your balance.

**What to do about it:**

*Regular movement* will prevent the joint from stiffening up and it will also feel less painful when you start to move if it hasn't had a chance to seize up in one position. Gentle exercise will not be damaging to an arthritic joint, even if it feels a bit sore to start with. As long as you are following what you feel and not forcing it into any positions, moving will be helpful.

*Strengthening exercises* for the muscles around the joint. Most joints rely on the muscles around them for support, but if a joint is painful, you are less likely to move it, so the muscles can weaken quite quickly. There are many variations of exercises which can be suitable, but it is important that you are assessed and then advised by a professional who can give you the exercises that are right for you.

*Find a practitioner* who can give you treatment to release the soft tissue around the joint and take the strain off it, to allow for a reduction in inflammation and to prevent worsening of the arthritis.

For ways to treat your joint pain and tension, please look at chapter 7 on page 79.

## Plantar fasciitis

The plantar fascia is the strong membrane on the sole of your foot that holds everything in its place. 'Itis' means inflammation of, so plantar fasciitis is inflammation of the membrane under your foot.

The main symptom is pain, either in the heel or spreading under the foot or up into the Achilles tendon. The pain is particularly bad when you put weight on your foot first thing in the morning or after sitting for a time. In relatively mild cases, the pain wears off once you have started walking. My patients often describe having to hobble to the bathroom in the middle of the night or in the morning but being able to walk normally after that.

Some people also develop bone spurs on their heel, which are small extra growths of bone that gradually develop in response to the irritation caused by chronic inflammation in the plantar fascia. While they are not themselves painful, they do cause pain in the surrounding tissues.

In my experience, the inflammation that starts this condition is caused by tightness in the muscles attaching into the sole of your foot. This is linked to tightness in the muscles in your upper leg, which tense up because the bones of your pelvis are rotated. I have successfully treated many people with plantar fasciitis without ever touching their feet. If you find and treat the cause of the problem, your body is normally able to heal the area of pain by completing the inflammatory cycle. For more information about this, please see chapter 3 on page 27.

Find a therapist who can assess and correct your pelvic alignment.

## Repetitive strain injury

Repetitive strain injury (RSI) is a general term used to describe the pain felt in muscles, nerves and tendons caused by repetitive movement and overuse.[7]

It mainly affects your neck, shoulders and arms and can produce symptoms such as pain, stiffness, swelling, numbness, tingling and weakness. It is caused by activities that are repetitive and of a high intensity over a long period, or in an awkward position that forces into a poor posture. It is also known to get worse with vibrations, in the cold, or if you are stressed.

The most important thing that you can do is to identify the trigger of your RSI, remembering that there may be more than one. If the cause is work-related, your employer has a duty to provide you with the correct equipment and work conditions to prevent incidents of RSI when reasonably possible. Making changes to the things that you spend all day doing will take the strain off your body and help it to heal the inflammation that has built up.

There are suggestions of how you can treat specific joints in chapter 7 on page 79.

## Rotator cuff injury

The rotator cuff is a group of muscles that wrap around your shoulder, keeping the joint in place and stable while allowing a wide range of movement. The tendons of these muscles can become inflamed due to overuse (stress from restrictions elsewhere in your body), or wear and tear.

Symptoms include a dull ache, pain on movement and weakness in the muscles. If you have had an injury to your shoulder, it is important to seek medical attention to make sure you don't need any immediate treatment.

As with frozen shoulder, finding and treating the cause is the long-term solution. The self-treatment techniques shown in chapter 7 will help you to manage the symptoms in the shorter term.

## Scar tissue

A scar is your body's way of replacing tissue that has been removed or damaged. It does this by laying down extra collagen fibres in the area as part of the healing process. This is an essential reaction, but scars can cause long-term problems for some people.

The scar that you get on your skin from an injury or operation is very obvious and you will be very aware of it if it is too tight or not healing properly. What is not so easy to detect is the internal scarring that occurs wherever tissue has been changed or disturbed. Sometimes, particularly after abdominal surgery, adhesions can form. These are bands of scar tissue that form between the scar tissue and organs, which can result in chronic pain and problems such as infertility. When excessive scarring occurs following joint surgery, it will cause pain and stiffness long after the expected recovery time.

Any deep scars will alter your posture, strength and flexibility in the local area, but they also have the potential to do the same in other areas of your body.

There are many products on the market that claim to reduce visible scarring; my opinion is that the more natural the product, the more likely it is to be able to work with your body to result in changes.

Internal scarring is more problematic, but if you are aware of the potential for post-operative problems, they are less likely to occur. Discussing it with your surgeon before the operation is advisable, so that they can tell you what the risks are and what they and you can do to minimise them. After the operation you can help yourself by doing the prescribed exercises, drinking plenty of water and trying to move as normally as possible.

If you are able to have gentle bodywork such as myofascial release, it will safely encourage the scar tissue fibres to lay down in the right direction, which makes them less likely to cause problems in the future. No treatment can eliminate scars, but their effects can be altered.

It is hard to give you specific advice on how to help problems caused by scars, as they are so individual. But in my experience, it is possible to reduce their effects and the on-going symptoms that they are causing. Chapter 7 on page 79 has a description of how you can treat your own scars.

## Surgery

Recovery from surgery very much depends on whether it was planned or was an emergency; where it was; how it was performed; and the severity of the condition. Please make sure that you follow whatever advice you have been given by your medical professionals.

However, there are some common factors that you can control to some extent, which may help your recovery:

- Ensuring that you are well hydrated is very important for every system of your body.
- Breathing to control your pain and reduce anxiety can make a big difference.
- Listening to your body as you are healing is vital – moving little and often can prevent stiffness from building up.

Chapter 5 on page 57 has much more information on these factors.

## Tendonitis

'Itis' means inflammation, so tendonitis is simply inflammation of a tendon. Tendons are the strong bands that attach each end of your muscles to bone. They are vulnerable to injury and inflammation because they are not very stretchy and do not have a very good blood supply.

This means that if they are injured, for example by being overstretched, twisted or suffering a direct blow, it takes much longer for them to heal. Tendonitis also occurs when stress is put onto the tendon from tightness and restrictions elsewhere in your body. For instance, if your pelvis is rotated, the forces transmitted through your fascial network will put your muscles and tendons under tension. So even if there is a minor injury, the tendon is much more likely to overstretch and become inflamed. This may happen without an actual injury if the irritation from other restrictions is bad enough.

Tendonitis can occur in any muscles, but the most common places are shoulders (rotator cuff), elbows (tennis and golfer's elbow) and ankles (Achilles tendonitis).

### *What to do about it:*

*Rest.* Your body needs time to heal, and the inflammatory response is its way of doing that. If you keep doing the things that are aggravating your tendon injury, your body will not have a chance to do its job and it will delay healing. There will always be jobs that have to be done, but if it is possible to get help or do them slower or in a different way than usual, you will be out of pain quicker and less likely to suffer the long-term problems of chronic inflammation.

*Gentle movement.* It is important to keep moving to avoid the area becoming stiff. Common sense needs to be applied here! Don't worry about moving the area but do not push into pain.

For ways to treat yourself please look at chapter 7 on page 79.

## References

1. https://cks.nice.org.uk/topics/back-pain-low-without-radiculopathy/background-information/prevalence/ Accessed 30th October 2022.

2. N. E. Foster, J. R. Anema, D. Cherkin, R. Chou, S. P. Cohen, D. P. Gross, P. H. Ferreira, et al. *"Prevention and Treatment of Low Back Pain: Evidence, Challenges, and Promising Directions."* Lancet 391, no. 10137 (2018): 2368–83.

3. G. Liptan, S. Mist, C. Wright, A. Arzt, and K. D. Jones. *"A Pilot Study of Myofascial Release Therapy Compared to Swedish Massage in Fibromyalgia."* Journal of Bodywork and Movement Therapies 17, no. 3 (2013): 365–70.

4. https://www.incontinence.co.uk/what-percentage-of-the-population-are-affected-by-incontinence Accessed 30th October 2022.

5. https://www.nhs.uk/conditions/coronavirus-covid-19/long-term-effects-of-coronavirus-long-covid/ Accessed 30th October 2022.

6. https://www.floridamedicalclinic.com/blog/what-is-the-mind-body-connection/ Accessed 6th November 2022.

7. https://www.nhs.uk/conditions/repetitive-strain-injury-rsi/ Accessed 30th October 2022.

## CHAPTER 5

# SIMPLE STEPS TO WORKING WITH YOUR BODY

*Please remember that the advice given in this chapter is general in nature and if you require individual advice, you should consult your own therapist.*

## Drink enough water

### Did you know ...

About 60% of your body is made of water and most of that water is inside your cells. In fact, two thirds of your cells' volume is made up of water.

It is really important to stay well hydrated because every system in your body needs water to work properly.

### What happens when you drink more water?

- Your joints are better lubricated, which allows them to move more freely and not stiffen up so easily. This can make a difference even if you already have wear and tear in a joint.

- Your digestion improves as your body needs water to absorb the nutrients from food. Water also helps movement through your digestive tract, so it will help reduce constipation.

- All your cells can work more efficiently. They need water for all the chemical reactions that must happen for your body to stay healthy.

- Your muscles are looser and more flexible when you move and exercise, so they can get stronger without being damaged.

## *What if you get dehydrated?*

There are some warning signs that should let you know that you are becoming dehydrated:

- Urine is a darker colour than normal.
- Low volume of urine.
- Very thirsty.
- Reduced concentration.
- Headache.
- Dizziness.
- Tired or sleepy.
- Dry mouth.
- Dry skin.

Not drinking just because you don't have enough time, or you are worried about not being able to get to a toilet, is not a good idea. Some changes that happen in your body when you are dehydrated are:

- Your joints and muscles become tighter and less flexible, which can lead to them feeling stiff and sore. Any problems that you have can feel worse, simply because you need to drink more.
- You are at increased risk of getting a urinary tract infection (UTI).
- Cells can become damaged, which affects their ability to work properly. This can lead to your physical and mental performance suffering.
- Your body can't control your temperature, heart rate or blood pressure properly, which can make you feel ill and can be very dangerous.

## *How to help yourself:*

Make sure that you drink enough.

- The European Food Safety Authority recommends that each day, women should drink about 1.6 litres and men should drink about 2.0 litres of fluid.[1]

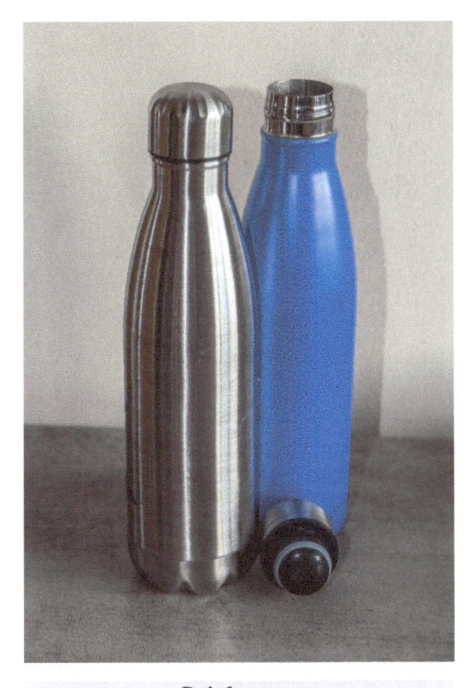

*Drink water*

- The amount that you need to drink at a particular time depends on your size, temperature and activity levels.
- Any liquids that you drink count towards the total, but the recommended amounts are on top of any water that you might be getting from the food that you eat.
- All drinks provide water, but if you are drinking anything other than plain water, remember that your drink will also have other ingredients, which may include sugar.
- Sipping your drinks slowly throughout the day is better than drinking a lot in one go.
- It is possible to drink too much water. If your urine is very pale and you are passing a lot of urine frequently then you may be too hydrated.

Remember that healthy cells lead to a healthy body.

## Breathe properly

Strange as it sounds, there is a right and wrong way of breathing. Many people breathe in the wrong way for their whole lives, and don't get any major problems. But if you already have an underlying condition or are in pain a lot of the time, the way that you breathe can have a big effect on the rest of your body.

If you have a history of breathing problems such as asthma, chronic obstructive pulmonary disease (COPD), pneumonia or chest infections, you may already be aware of how difficult it is to take in a full breath of air when you are tight, coughing or in pain.

Bruised and fractured ribs are extremely painful due to the large number of nerve endings around your ribs, and because they are moved every time you breathe. The pain from these injuries tends to last for many weeks and your body will very quickly get used to trying to avoid movement in the injured area by bracing and taking shallower breaths.

If you have ever been winded in a fall, you will know exactly what it feels like to have the breath knocked out of you. As we discussed in chapter 3, the impact of the fall itself causes your body to tighten up and freeze, and that applies to your diaphragm and chest area, too. If it is never released, you continue to breathe in a way that compensates for that tightness. How many times have you been winded?

## What happens when you don't breathe properly?

If you are not breathing in as much oxygen as you need, and not breathing out enough carbon dioxide, your brain will make you breathe faster until the levels are back to where they should be. This can happen when you are exercising, too cold, stressed or in pain. But if you aren't breathing in the right way, it will occur more often. This can lead to you feeling very tired and short of breath and tense and achy in your upper back and across your shoulders. It also makes pain, tension or anxiety worse and harder to cope with.

If your diaphragm is tight and not working efficiently, you will end up overusing your accessory breathing muscles. These are muscles that are located around your chest and shoulders, and they shouldn't normally be used much in breathing. When they have to take over, they will tighten up and cause pain and tension in your upper back and chest.

## How should you breathe?

The diaphragm and intercostal muscles between your ribs are the main muscles that should be working when you breathe in. Your diaphragm is a dome shaped muscle that attaches all the way round the bottom of your ribs, in front of your spine and across the centre of your body. Your oesophagus (food pipe), aorta (large artery) and vena cava (large vein) pass through the muscle as it separates the top and bottom halves of your body.

When you contract your diaphragm, it flattens, pulling your lungs down and pushing your abdominal contents out. This increases the volume of your lungs, decreasing the pressure and allowing air to be drawn in.

That is why diaphragmatic breathing is sometimes called belly breathing.

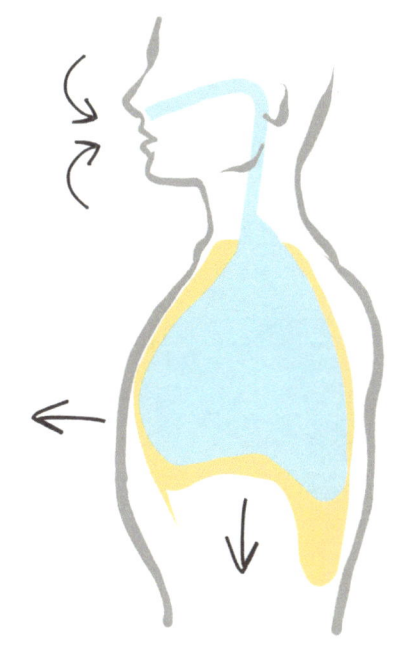

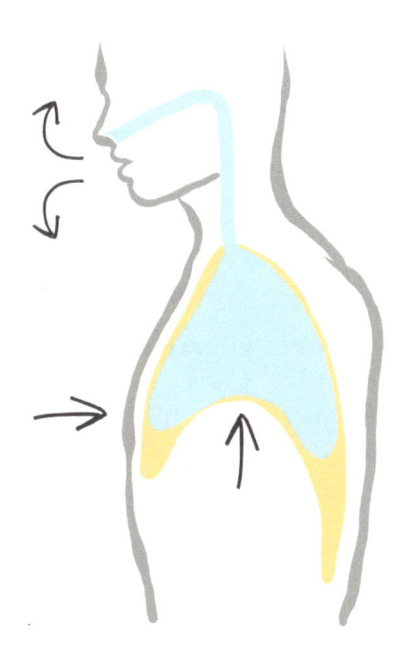

Breathing in                                    Breathing out

*Breathing*

Breathing out shouldn't take any effort at all; by relaxing your diaphragm or settling your belly back in, the volume of your lungs will decrease, increasing the pressure and pushing the air back out. But remember to give yourself time to empty your lungs, so that they are not full of stale air when you try to take the next breath in. One of the problems when people hyperventilate is that they are trying so hard to take the next breath, they don't allow themselves to breathe out first.

You won't get it right all the time, as it takes practice to form the right habits and to retrain your muscles, so you don't have to think about what you are doing. Just give yourself a few minutes every day to focus on it, and your breathing will improve. It's a good idea to practice diaphragmatic breathing in different positions and situations so that it's a more realistic scenario. For example, waiting at lights in the car, standing to do the washing up or lying in bed.

### *How to help yourself:*

As soon as you feel that you are breathing faster or using your shoulders more than your diaphragm for breathing in, focus on breathing properly until it settles down again.

An easy way to tell if you are doing diaphragmatic breathing is to gently place one hand on your belly, just below your ribs.
As you take a breath in your hand should move up and out, sinking back down when you breathe out. Your shoulders shouldn't be moving much at all when you do this – if they do, just soften them and try again.

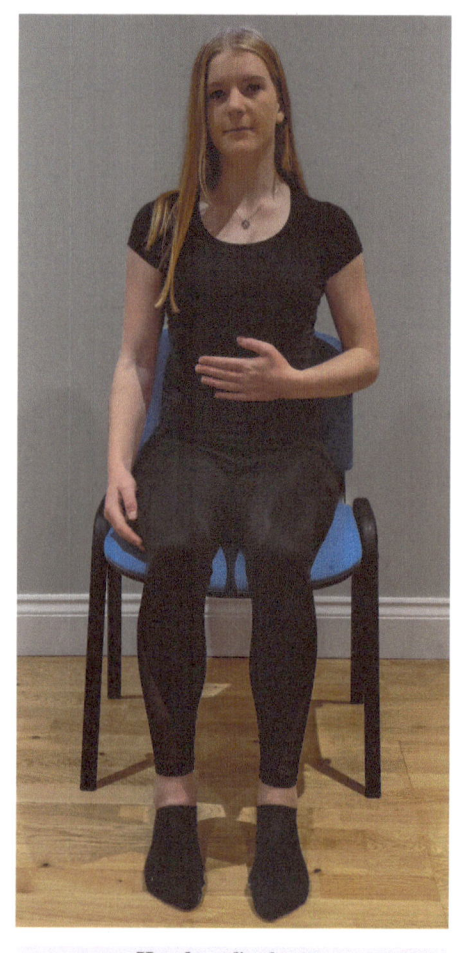

**Hand on diaphragm**

If you are in pain whenever you move, the natural response is to tense up and hold your breath. This makes the pain worse, and you probably end up feeling very tense and stressed. So, if you expect it to hurt, breathe in before you start moving and slowly blow the breath out with your movement. You may need to do this in several stages to get to where you need to be, but that's okay. The main thing is focussing on breathing out and letting go of the muscles that don't need to be working. Don't take very deep breaths in each time though, or you may hyperventilate.

## Stretch

Don't stretch, release!

Have you ever watched a cat or dog stretch? They make it look like one of the most self-indulgent, luxurious, pleasurable activities in the world. And so it should be.

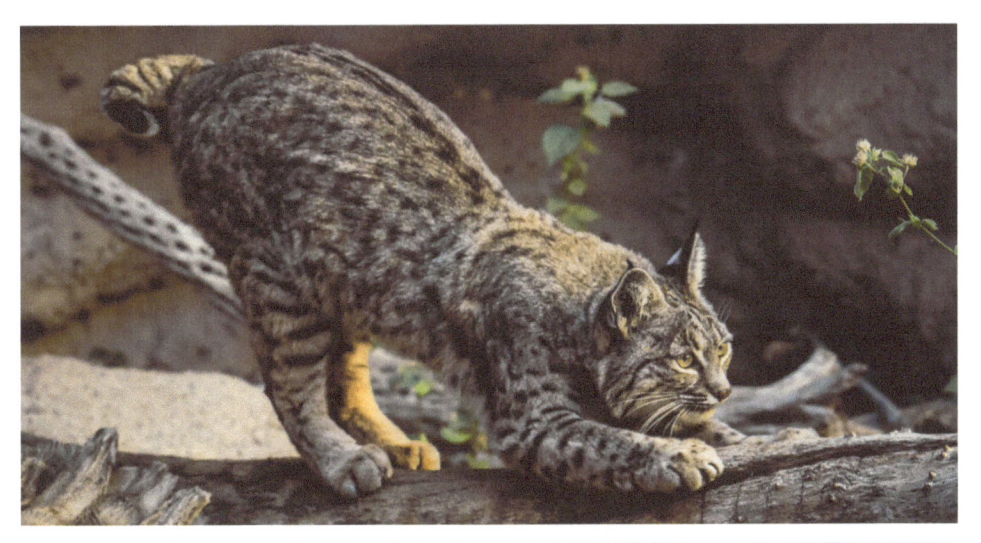

*Stretching – Photograph courtesy of @PeteMecozziPhotography via Twenty20*

Now think about when you woke up this morning. When you first began to move and your body began to stretch out, was that the moment that you got up, had a shower, sorted out the family, and started your day?

Imagine how it would feel to give your body just two minutes to be self-indulgent and luxurious before you get out of bed, so as your muscles wake up, they have the opportunity to open out and release the tension that has been building up overnight. Then, once you get out of bed, your body is prepared and better able to meet the demands put on it.

Your morning stretch and the stretches that follow a good yawn will change each time, depending on where in your body needs to open up. You don't need to know what to do, just trust your body and follow its need to stretch.

But there are times when you do need to think about stretching a specific muscle or area of your body – for example, before and after exercise, or if you have an injury or painful condition. This is when it is very important to do it correctly, otherwise the stretch will be ineffective or even cause damage.

### Why do you feel tight?

When your body is loose, relaxed and elastic, it can move and change with you. But it is very common to gradually feel tighter – this is often put down to getting older, but it isn't inevitable.

As the pressure builds up in your muscles and they stiffen up, they gradually get thicker and shorter. This means that the blood flow isn't as good as it should be to help with healing, so you get more scarring, with makes the area even stiffer.

Some of the reasons for feeling tight are dehydration, poor posture, weakness in a different part of your body, not exercising properly, overusing muscles, and stress.

Remember that where you feel your symptoms is often different to where the cause of them is. Your tightness may be due to problems in another part of your body and is your body's way of compensating and trying to protect itself. So, there is no point in simply stretching the tight bit without also finding and treating the cause.

Stretching opens up the layers of your muscles, which helps the blood flow. It takes the pressure off the nerves, so pain and inflammation can be prevented or improved.

### How to help yourself:

Give yourself time to stretch in the mornings and during the day. Whenever you notice that your muscles are becoming tight or restless, have a yawn and go with your body. Why not try now?

- Slowly open up to the point where you can feel the stretch but there is no pain.

- Hold there – NEVER STRETCH INTO PAIN. Your body's response to pain is to pull back, so it will make things tighter.
- Wait at that point until you feel the muscle release and get longer. If you don't wait for that change, you won't have stretched.
- Remember that each time you do a stretch, even to the same muscle, its requirements will be different. One day it might release after 30 seconds and the next day it might take 5 minutes.

Chapter 7 on page 79 includes lots of different ways that you can help yourself to improve your posture and reduce symptoms. But they are just suggestions. Once you get used to feeling what your body needs, you don't necessarily need to stick to stretching in a certain position. As long as you follow the principles, you will do no harm to yourself, and you will be able to identify and release tension before it has a chance to build up and cause more problems.

Yoga and Pilates classes are increasingly popular for people who want to have guidance on exercising and stretching safely. There are many different approaches within both disciplines, all of which have a place in the market, but it can get confusing. I would recommend using a teacher who has training and experience in teaching people who have pain, as otherwise you may end up doing movements that are not good for you.

Finding a teacher and approach that suit you are very important factors, as you are more likely to be motivated and want to attend the classes regularly. Small classes are generally a good idea so that the teacher has a good view of how you are moving and is able to correct you quickly if needed.

Whichever class you take, the rules of stretching still apply. If your teacher is not willing to let you go at your own pace, please find someone else who is.

## Listen to your body

Don't wait for pain. Most of the time your body starts to tighten up a long time before the pain starts in response to activities. This is its way of trying to protect itself from overuse and injury, and if you respond to it straight away, it will relax again once the perceived danger has passed. However, if you continue to do the same thing, the danger signals will escalate, and your body will have to try harder and harder to get you to stop. If you ignore the tension, it will start hurting, and if you ignore that too, then expect a muscle spasm or cramp to stop you.

Animals are the masters of listening to their bodies and not just when it comes to stretching. Can you imagine your cat, dog or horse staying in a position or continuing a movement that does not feel right or is painful? And there is absolutely no reason why we should, but we do!

If you are willing to be flexible in how you move and work, your nervous system can relax, and it will gradually become less irritable and allow you to get away with doing more. Planning activities so that you can change the height, angle, and timings to suit your body will give you that flexibility and save you a lot of suffering. Remember that just because you have always done something in a certain way, doesn't mean it has to stay that way.

'I'll just finish this…'

How often do you think that and half an hour later find yourself in exactly the same position, doing the same thing?

Whether the thing you are doing is computer work, gardening, housework or knitting, it is very easy to get so absorbed in your task that it is difficult to listen to the signals that your body is sending you.

Another common factor in symptom flare-ups is focussing on the amount of work or exercise that has to be done. So, deciding in advance that you are going to swim 30 lengths, cut all the hedges back, play all 18 holes of golf, is putting a lot of pressure onto yourself to achieve that level of activity.

Whether or not you have a condition that causes pain, tightness or fatigue, if you don't listen to your body, you will cause an increase in tension that over time will lead to symptoms.

If you do have an underlying condition, it is even more important to listen to your body and pace yourself according to how you are feeling at that time on that day. It is normal for symptoms to vary from day to day, so you will find that your activity levels will vary accordingly.

## *How to help yourself:*

Take time to be aware of your body, particularly joints and muscles, during activities that you spend a lot of your day doing. Can you feel areas tightening up after a certain length of time?

This increased awareness of the changes that gradually occur during the day allows you to work with your body and better manage your symptoms, or even prevent them from building up.

Often, before you feel pain during an activity you get tightness. But if your whole body is always tight, it is very hard to detect these early warning signs.

Myofascial release treatment can help your body to untangle so that it becomes the norm to feel loose and flexible, rather than tight.

Then it is much easier to detect the early warning signs and do something about them before they lead to a flare up of spasm, inflammation and pain. There is more information about this treatment in chapter 8 on page 111.

So rather than starting an activity by setting yourself targets of how long or how many you are going to do, try doing it until you are aware that your body is starting to react. This takes practice, patience and concentration to begin with, but it does get easier.

Remember that the level of activity you are able to do before you need to stop or change will vary day by day – that is normal.

When you do feel that your body isn't happy with what you are doing, stop! Then either rest or change what you are doing to a different activity, alter your position or stretch before you carry on.

Ask for help. It doesn't mean that you are giving in or admitting defeat. If you overdo it, you will need more help for longer than if you follow your body.

If a task feels overwhelming, try to break it down into stages. This even applies to something as simple as carrying a box into a different room. Plan where you can take a rest. Before you start, clear surfaces along the way so that you have somewhere safe to put it down. Have a chair waiting for you when you have finished.

## Posture

In the following list I have picked out just a few of the activities that can cause postural problems that I see every day in my patients. If they apply to you, looking at the positions that you spend most of your time in will be helpful.

- Driving

What sort of driver are you? If you are nervous, do your shoulders end up round your ears after a stressful journey? Do the other road users wind you up, making your own tension worse?

I always ask my patients what makes their symptoms worse, and driving is one of the more common replies. Cars these days are much better for your body than they used to be, but only if you know how to set them up correctly to meet your body's needs.

Some things to check and adjust in your car (apart from the mirror) are the steering wheel height, seat height and position, lumbar support, and head rest position. Heated seats are also a great way of keeping your back relaxed when you are driving.

- Walking dogs

Unless your dog is perfect at walking to heel at all times, you will probably have experienced that sudden pull up your arm and into your shoulder as he discovers a scent in the opposite direction that has to be investigated.

The first thing to try to do is soften your body and follow him – unless he is about to pull you off your feet. The natural reaction to a sudden change in pull or direction is to brace yourself, but that is when a lot of the damage can occur. By staying centred and feeling what direction he is heading for, it is much easier to predict movements and to stay with them. Your body won't be as vulnerable to injury, as you will be more able to go with the pull.

- Carrying shopping

Even if you only have to load and unload your shopping bags from the car, it can take a toll on your back. Planning ahead and taking your time can save you from future pain and injury. The main thing is to split your shopping into smaller, more manageable sized bags – that doesn't mean you can carry more bags at one time, though!

Be aware of your limits and be prepared to do more trips into the house with fewer bags or ask for help.

- Staying in the same position all day

Whatever your job or hobbies, your body will react to the positions that you spend a lot of time in. My patients who teach young children and spend most of the day bent over, all have back pain. Surgeons, dentists and vets get pain and tension in their neck and across their shoulders from the position in which they stay when they are operating.

The way to look after your body is to change position as soon as you become aware of the tension increasing, and before the pain sets in. Only you will know how to get around the problem, but it is very important that you do find a solution so that your pain doesn't stop you working, exercising or being able to enjoy your hobbies.

Chapter 7 on page 79 shows some ways that you can treat yourself to improve your posture.

### References

1. European Food Safety Authority (EFSA) Panel on Dietetic Products, Nutrition, and Allergies. *"Scientific Opinion on Dietary Reference Values for Water."* EFSA Journal 8, no. 3 (2010). doi:10.2903/j.efsa.2010.1459.

> *No matter how far down the wrong road you have gone, turn around.*

John F. Barnes

# CHAPTER 6

# EVERYDAY WAYS TO HELP YOURSELF

*As with all the advice that I give in this book, it is very important to follow what you feel and to stop if what you are doing makes any symptoms worse or if it doesn't feel right. It could be that you need to receive a course of hands-on treatment to help existing conditions before you are able to follow these suggestions. That would be worth doing, as once you are balanced and not in pain all the time, it will be much easier to do things properly.*

## Lifting

Learning how to lift and move heavy objects safely is essential. Following this advice will not only help to prevent injuries but will allow you to use your body in a kind way, so your muscles don't have to tighten up to protect themselves.

### How to lift safely

1} Think before you start to lift. Take a minute to look at where you will be moving the load to. Is there a clear path from where you will be starting, or are there obstructions? Will you need help either to lift it in the first place or once you get there? Is there a place to rest if you need to change your grip or if you are struggling?

2} Hold the load close to your waist. Keeping the load close to your waist will reduce the amount of pressure on your back. Hold the heaviest side next to your body and try to move it as close to you as possible before trying to lift it.

3} Check that you have a stable position.
Your feet should be placed comfortably apart with one leg slightly further forward to help with your balance. Remember, you may need to shift the position of your feet during the lift to stay stable. If you are wearing unsuitable footwear it will make this much more difficult.

4} Make sure you have a good grip on the load.
Depending on the size of the load relative to the length of your arms, you may need to make a few adjustments to your grip before you start the lift. If you do need to change your grip, put the load down first. This might be the time to ask for help if you can feel that your grip isn't firm enough.

5} Don't bend your back when you are lifting.
Your spine shouldn't be perfectly straight as it naturally curves slightly in at the bottom, out in the middle and in again at your neck. But if you bend forward to lift, it puts enormous pressure on your back and that is when injuries occur. At the start of the lift, bend your knees and hips, sticking your bottom out if needed, to get down to the same level as the load.

6} Keep your back in a good position while you are lifting. Keep your hips and knees bent while you are starting to raise the load up and bring it close into your body before straightening your legs again.

7} Don't twist when you lift.
Avoid twisting your back or leaning sideways – keep your shoulders level and facing the same direction as your hips. When you change direction, step around so your whole body follows your feet instead of turning your upper body.

8} Look ahead of you.
Once you have lifted the load, try not to look down, as this will start to bend

your back too. This is why checking that the path is clear before you start is a good idea.

9} Move smoothly.
Keep your movements slow and controlled so you can feel what the load and your body are doing. Then if there is a problem you will have more chance of making adjustments to correct it or of putting the load down safely.

10} Know your limits.
Just because you are able to lift something, doesn't mean you should lift it! The lifting we are talking about here is part of the daily, repetitive jobs that need doing, not just a one-off load. That makes a massive difference to the strain that is put on your body and is what is likely to lead to problems. If you are in doubt, please get help.

11} Don't bend your back when putting the load down. Having lifted the load with a perfect posture, moved your feet and controlled your movements, please don't then hurt yourself by putting it down without thinking. You need to do the same bending of the hips and knees, sticking your bottom out as when you lifted it up. Get your feet as close as possible to where you will be placing the load and try not to stick your chin forward as you put it down.

## Gardening

1} Check your tools.
Are you using the right tool for the job? Are the tools the right size for you? Are all the tools in good working order?

2} Wheelbarrows.
Does your wheelbarrow have a flat tyre, or a broken handle? Using a wheelbarrow that is broken immediately puts a strain on your whole body, as you have to work so much harder to keep it upright and to wheel it in a straight line. Then you load it (or overload it), and it all goes wrong. To protect your back and shoulders, only use a wheelbarrow that is in good working order and never

put too much into it. When you are pushing a loaded wheelbarrow, try to keep your shoulders relaxed and look straight ahead. Lift the handles enough so that you do not have to bend your back to reach them.
If you feel that your back is tightening up, have a rest.

3} Listen to your body.
As soon as you become aware that any muscles are starting to tighten up, you need to stop what you are doing. But that does not necessarily mean abandoning the job altogether. You could take a quick break to stretch the part of you that you are feeling your symptoms in, or swap to a different task. For example, stop forking up and do a bit of sweeping or empty the wheelbarrow. Basically, your body does not like repetitive movements, so if you continue to do the same thing, ignoring the warning signs, your body will gradually get tighter and tighter and then more and more painful until you are forced to stop. Afterwards, you are likely to have a flare up of existing problems or overstretch and injure yourself. If you can get your head round working in this way, following what your body is telling you instead of fighting it, life will become much less painful.

4} Check your posture.
Do you look down most of the time when you are gardening? As I said in chapter 4 page on page 35, your head is very heavy, so looking down will drag your upper body forwards, causing tension and pain in your upper back. Maintaining a good core position and glancing downwards when you need to is the best way.

5} Sweeping.
This is a repetitive job that causes a lot of pain, even for people who do not have a back problem. Check the length of the handle, make sure there are no broken bits and look at the head of the broom to ensure that it is up to the job. Sorry for repeating myself, but this is so important that I am

going to: do not look down or bend your back. Do look ahead and stand with your feet pointing in the direction you are moving with the opposite leg to the broom further forward. Transfer your weight from one leg to another as you move forwards and backwards, instead of leading with your arms. Hold the broom with your hands high enough up to feel comfortable in your shoulders and back.

6} Switch to a different task when you become aware of any tension building up. Normally this will be felt between your shoulder blades or in your lower back, but the reason for it is pulling from the front of your body.

## Technology

- Computer work

Whether you work at a computer all day or just use it at home in the evenings, the way that your screen, keyboard, and chair are set up will have a very real and ongoing effect on your body.

People tend to get fixed in the same position after a while, particularly if they are concentrating hard or under pressure to get a piece of work done. As I am typing this, I can feel my shoulders starting to tense up – time to get up for a glass of water and remember to keep breathing!

Your employer should assist you in getting the right equipment to be able to sit and work without pain, but if you are using your computer at home, it's up to you to look after yourself.

Your seat should have good lumbar support (at the bottom of your back) and have adjustable height and tilt. If you need to reach to different areas regularly, having wheels and the ability to pivot is helpful.

Using a footrest, even for part of the day, can help to change your position and prevent your body from getting stuck in one position. If the height of the footrest can be changed too, that is even better.

Adjustable height desks and workstations are becoming more popular and are ideal if you struggle to sit for a long time.

Check the levels of your screen, keyboard, and mouse. They should all be comfortable for you to use without straining. Remember that if you share your desk with someone else, you will need to recheck your setup each time you sit down to work.

- Laptops

Laptops should not be used on your lap!

As soon as you start to work from that position, your whole body is forced into flexion, putting stress and strain on your neck, back and wrists in particular. By placing your laptop on a table, preferably using all the same advice as for computer work, you will be much more comfortable and prevent many problems in the future.

- Mobile phones and tablets

We are increasingly dependent on having access to technology wherever we are. The main issue with this is the posture that your body is pulled into as soon as you look down and use both hands to type and hold the device.

If you're not sure what that is, try it now and focus on the changes in tension that you feel happening all over your body.

Some solutions are to limit the time that you spend focussing on your phone or tablet, or at least place it on a table in front of you (ideally tilted up) or sit in a chair that supports your back and arms so that you can hold it up comfortably in front of you.

- Holding phone between your ear and your shoulder

I know it is awkward having to do something with your hands and hold the phone at the same time but please don't do this. It immediately causes tension to build up in both sides of your neck and into your shoulders. If you do it for long periods of time or on a regular basis, it will be very difficult to release that tightness yourself and it will be very likely to result in pain and headaches.

Using the speaker phone option on your phone, or investing in a headset if you spend a lot of time talking on the phone, are both good ways to take the strain off your neck and prevent a build-up of pain.

## Babies and children

People tend to hold babies in the same arm and sit toddlers on the same hip every time they are carrying them. When this is coupled with the bent over posture that is normal when you are feeding a baby – either by breast or bottle – you can imagine the strain that it puts on your whole spine. As a rule, flexing and twisting at the same time is your back's worst nightmare and it will complain if you keep doing it, especially while carrying a wriggling child.

Try to alternate the sides that you are holding and carrying, staying aware of how you are lifting the baby or toddler up from the floor, chair, or cot. If you already have back pain, try sitting in a chair and asking your toddler to climb up onto your lap. Then it is much easier to get them into a good position and stand up.

If you are sitting to feed, pillows are the best way to support your arm while you support the baby. Sit well back into a comfortable chair with good lumbar positioning and place the pillows under your arm and across your lap to lay the baby on. Remembering to breathe and softening your neck and shoulders will also help.

> *Slow your breathing, quieten your mind and soften your body.*
>
> John F. Barnes

## CHAPTER 7

# TREATING YOURSELF

The techniques described in this section are based on John Barnes' Myofascial Release Approach®, which creates the conditions to allow your body to release restrictions that cause pain and tension.[1]

The focus is on releasing rather than strengthening, as the principles of myofascial release show us that it is essential to achieve the correct starting position before attempting to strengthen any weakness. A lot of the time, apparent weaknesses occur simply due to tension in the opposing muscle group.
I have treated athletes who go on to achieve personal bests in the days following their treatment. Their muscles cannot have become significantly bigger in that time, but by releasing the tension around a muscle, it is able to work much more efficiently straight away.

All the techniques that I am suggesting in this chapter are very gentle and should always be performed in a slow, controlled way. But sometimes you may have symptoms that are a sign of a more serious problem, that are related to something else going on in your body. Or your symptoms may simply be too irritable for the exercise that you are trying. So please make sure you only do what you feel confident with, and you stop immediately if you are unsure, if anything that you are doing doesn't feel right, or if your symptoms begin to get worse. If this does happen, it is best to get checked by a health professional or body worker before you do any more exercises. Remember that the advice given in this book is very general and cannot replace assessment and treatment from someone who can see and feel exactly what your specific problems are.

You may already know exercises or releases to help the problems that I describe here and of course if they help you, there is no reason to stop doing them.

However, you may find that these alternative suggestions are more practical for you.

There is always a reason for problems and remember that the cause may be in a different part of your body to the issue. The following examples are only a small selection of the numerous ways in which you can help yourself. The suggestions I have made are focussed on helping you to recognise and feel what is happening.

Research has shown that applying gentle, sustained pressure to an area for at least five minutes stimulates the body's anti-inflammatory response and so can speed healing.[2] Some of the advice given here is on how you can treat yourself using this method. Remember to go slowly and gently and to stop before you feel pain or if you experience any adverse effects.

## Feeling your body

Having noted where your issue is, the next step is to feel. This is surprisingly difficult when you have spent many years trying to ignore what your body is telling you so that it doesn't stop you from doing what you need to do. So, whether you are lying, standing or sitting, just take a moment to feel.

- Do you have pain anywhere?
- Where can you feel pockets or lines of tension?
- Is your weight going through both sides of your body evenly?
- How is your breathing?
- Are you bracing anywhere?

One way of feeling your body is to do a body scan. Imagine that a tiny version of you is inside your body and is able to travel anywhere. Starting with your toes, slowly move up your body, taking note of any areas that are tight or sore. You can pause in those places and just allow your breathing to slow and without any effort, soften the tension and experience any sensations.

Repeating this exercise when you are relaxed and not rushed will gradually make it easier to feel what is happening in your body. It will become much more obvious to you when something is causing your body to react. If you can feel, then you will be able to do something about the problem by changing the cause of it, not just forcing against it.

Remember that it doesn't matter how far you move into a position, just focus on what you feel. It is normal to move a different amount every time you do the same release, and both sides of your body are likely to move different amounts, too. If you know that you are a competitive person, try not to give yourself goals of how far or how much you are going to do. This approach may be frustrating to begin with, but once you learn how to feel and follow your body, you will be able to work with it and not against it. From here, your symptoms will become easier to manage and you will be able to prevent further problems in the future.

## How to treat yourself

### Using your hands

Gently place your hand over the affected area, allow it to sink into the skin and wait. No need to push or try to move anything; the warmth and pressure from your hand will also help your ground substance to thin and the fibres will start to release (as described in chapter 1 on page 7). Stop if it doesn't feel right, if it is uncomfortable to maintain the position, or if it is painful.

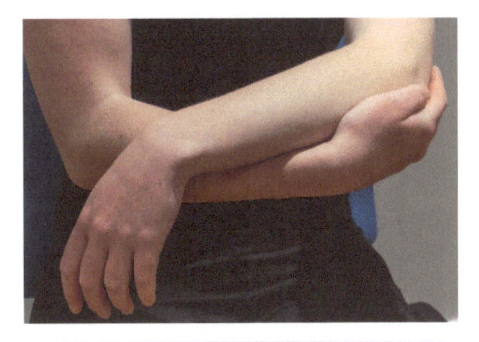

*Treating elbow*

### Using the contract/relax method

This way of exercising is very effective in helping you to feel where existing tightness is being held, and then being more able to let it go. As you have probably experienced, it is much easier to contract a tight muscle than to relax it when you need to. Rather than advising you to relax the tight area, I will show you how to tighten into it first, then hold for a count of ten and very slowly and gently allow it to soften and let go until it is limp and relaxed. Remember not to push into pain, though.

## Using a ball

Small balls such as tennis balls or Pilates balls can be used to access areas that are hard to reach with your hands. By using gentle, sustained pressure into tight areas, your body can release restrictions in the area. This shouldn't be painful, so if you find a point of pain, just move to the side of it with the ball.

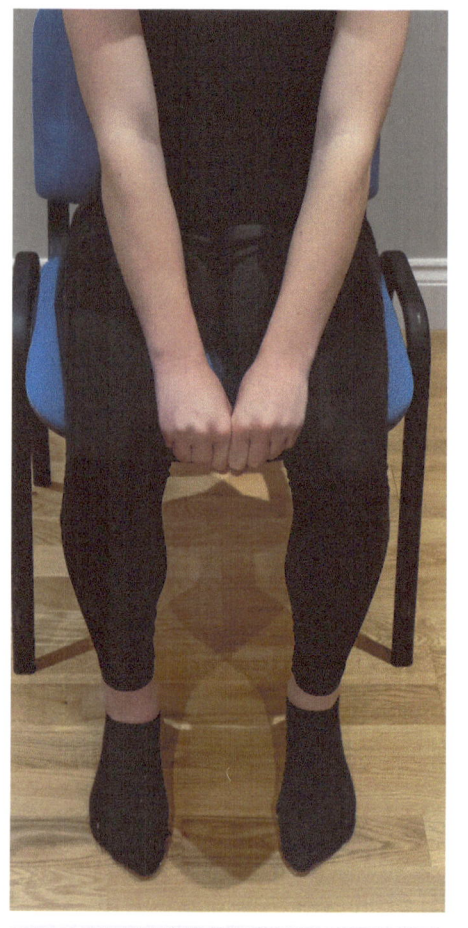

*Contract/relax*

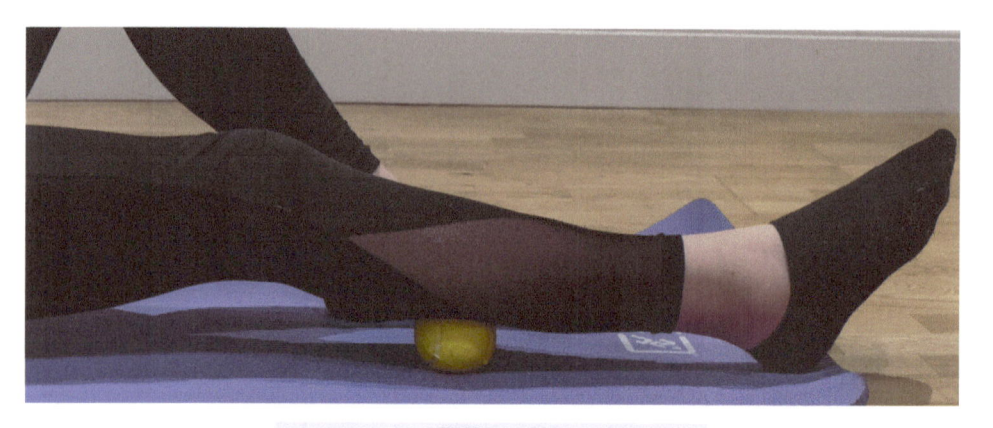

*Ball in calf*

## Using a foam roller

Foam rollers are lightweight foam cylinders that are used for deep tissue massage to help tight, painful muscles. You may have seen people vigorously rolling up and down on their foam roller, probably grimacing and quite possibly groaning in pain while they do it. Please do not roll on your roller! Research has shown that the effects of rolling on a foam roller on joint mobility is limited to ten minutes[3] and that it has the potential to cause tissue damage by the pressure that is exerted on the connective tissue, nerves, and blood vessels.[4]

The kinder and more effective way of using your foam roller is to lie or lean against it with the part of your body that you are trying to release. Then wait for at least five minutes to give your tissues a chance to change in response to the sustained pressure.

If you feel a release then it is fine to gently move into the next area of restriction that you feel, then wait again. In this way, you will not hurt yourself, as you are always following what you feel and not forcing any changes on your body.

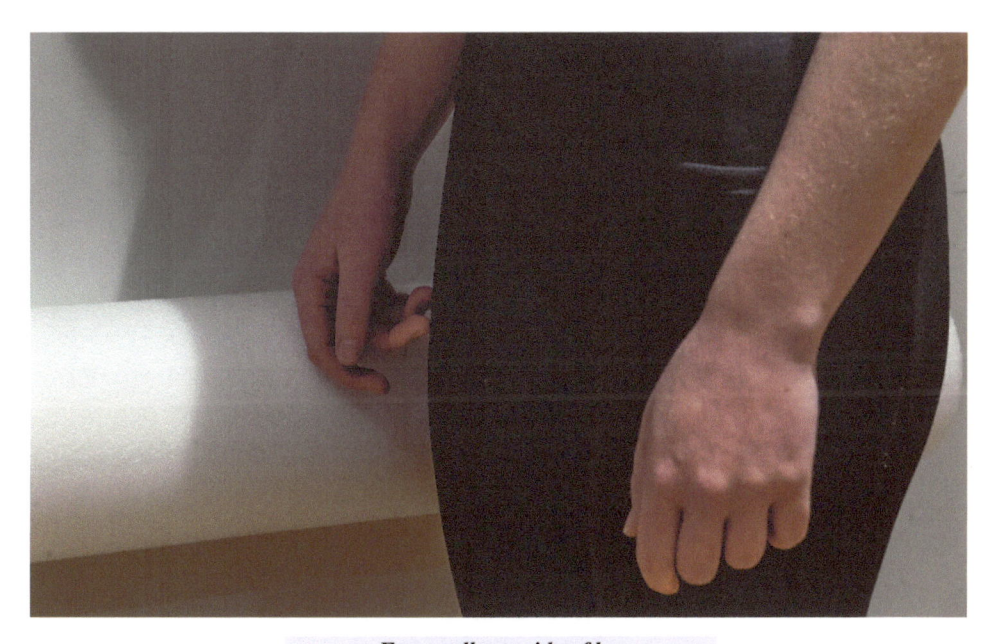

*Foam roller to side of leg*

If you don't feel a release, as long as you are comfortable you can stay in that position for as long as you need to. You may find that a different area of your body needs to change before the area you are working on. If this is the case, you can try scanning through your body to see if any other areas of discomfort or tension flag up. Then you can try to release there first. Remember that if your body has been compensating and building restrictions for years, it is unlikely to let everything go after one session of self-treatment.

### Things to remember

- Focus on what you feel as you move into each position until you feel a slight resistance (may be anywhere in your body).
- Hold at the barrier until you feel a release, for at least 3-5 minutes.
- Trust what you feel – follow your body.
- Never push into pain – remember that you are not trying to go as far as possible.
- If you experience an increase in your symptoms, STOP immediately.

### How to help scars

Place your hand on the skin over your scar, allowing the weight of your hand to rest down and wait. Over a few minutes, the warmth and pressure from your hand will start to release the tissues in and around the scar – chapter 8 on page 111 has all the details of how this works.

You will probably find that the skin around your scar goes soft much quicker than the scar itself, but just be patient and give the scar time to change – it will need regular treatments. You might find that your scar always feels a bit different, but it should be possible to make a difference. If you are seeing a therapist, ask them if there is anything specific you can do to help your scar, as I can only give very general advice here.
As always, stop straight away if what you are doing is making any symptoms worse.

## How to help your neck and upper back

### The front of your neck

This release is good for tension across your upper chest, which can cause pain into your neck and across your shoulders. It also helps to improve your posture if you tend to hold your chin forwards.

Place one hand skin on skin onto your sternum (breastbone) and allow the weight of your arm to gently hang down.

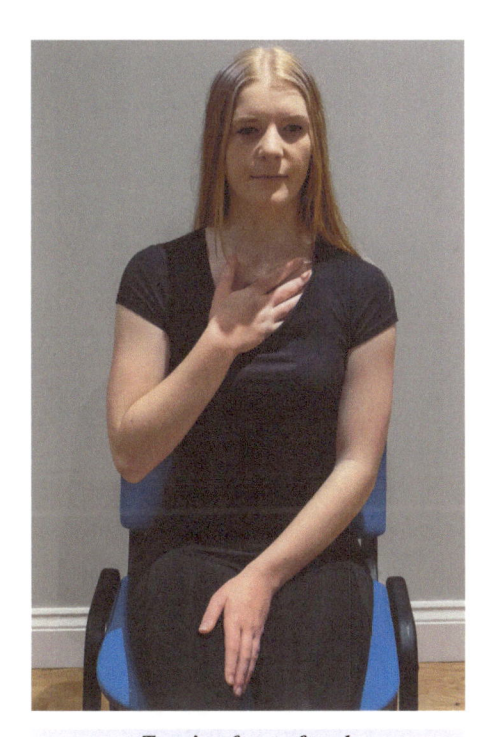

*Treating front of neck*

Allow your hand to sink in and follow any movements that you feel under your hand. Don't worry if you don't feel much; you will still be helping yourself by staying with it. If your head begins to move as you release, that is fine, but don't try to move it consciously. When you have finished, keep your hand in the same place until you have lifted your arm slightly, then very slowly peel your hand away. This can be done sitting or standing. Remember to breathe and aim to hold for a minimum of five minutes.

### Ball release for the back of your neck

This is a great way of softening the muscles that attach into the base of your skull. Try this for tension headaches too.

Position the ball at the back of your neck, just to the side of your spine. This can also be done with two balls at the same time, one on either side. Lean back onto the ball, slowly feeling it sink into your body until it meets resistance, then stop. Wait in that position, keeping the rest of your body soft and feel as your muscles open up.

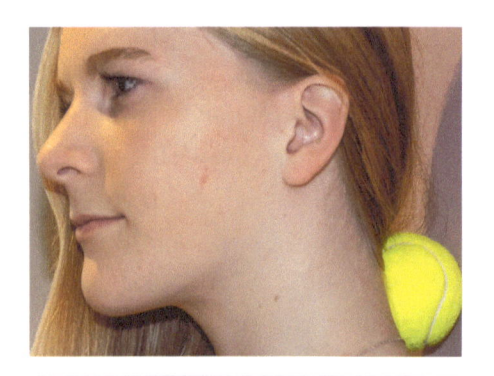

*Ball in back of neck*

For the best results, this release should take at least five minutes. If you are very sore, you should follow your body and stop if you need to. Remember that you are not looking to find the painful spots, just resistance. If the ball is on a point that is sore, try readjusting it so you are more comfortable. You could either do this release while standing and leaning against a wall, sitting in a high-backed chair, or lying on your back on the floor or bed.

## The side of your neck

Use this release when your shoulders are pulling up to your ears, and the muscles between your neck and shoulders (upper trapezius muscles) are tight and tender.

Place your hand skin on skin over the top of your opposite upper trapezius (the muscle that runs from the top of your shoulder to your neck) and allow gravity to take the weight of your arm.

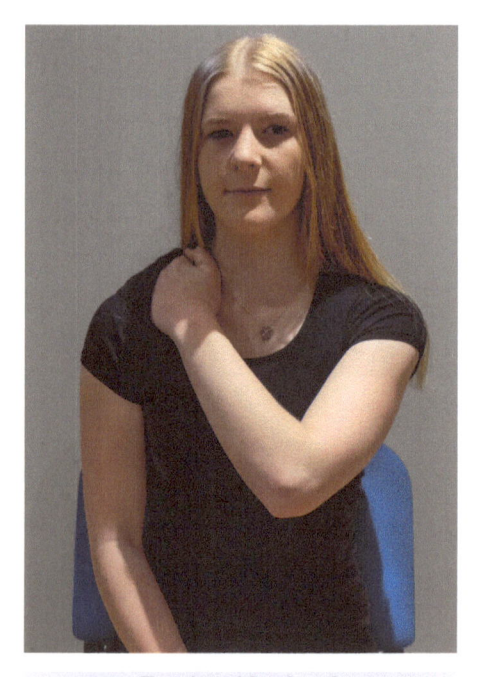

*Treating side of neck*

Allow your hand to sink in until you feel a release. When you have finished, keep your hand in the same place until you have lifted your arm slightly, then very slowly peel your hand away. Repeat on the opposite side (start with your best side). This can be done sitting or standing. Remember to breathe and aim to hold for a minimum of five minutes.

## How to help the middle of your back

### Side stretch

This will help to release tension on the side of your trunk and into your waist. If one of your shoulders sits lower than the other, it could be due to this tightness pulling it down, so this is a good release to try. Another reason for your shoulders to be at different levels could be that the higher side is being pulled up by tension in the muscle between your neck and shoulder. If this is the case, try the release for the side of your neck – the previous technique described in this chapter.

Grasp your wrist with the opposite hand. Pull your arm above your head and across your body, while actively elongating your body and wait for the release. Repeat on the other side if needed.

Try this in sitting and standing. The sitting release will focus more on your armpit and upper body. The standing release will focus on your lower body and possibly into your pelvis and hip.

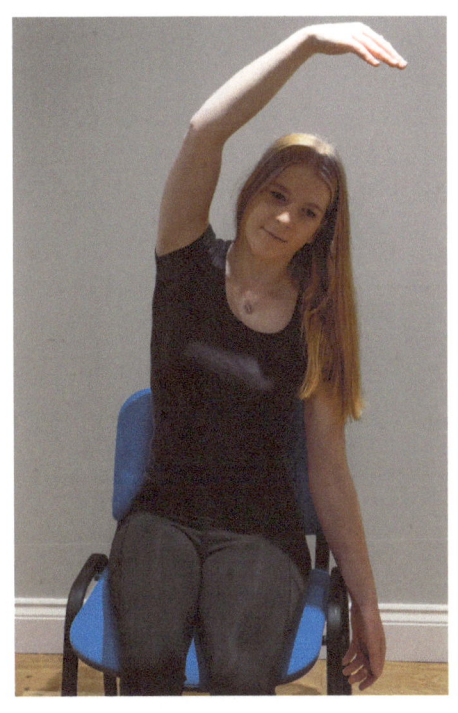

*Side stretch*

### Diaphragm release with foam roller

This is good to reduce tension in your mid and upper back. Your diaphragm tends to tighten up after you have been coughing a lot, and with stress, so if you feel you can't take a full deep breath, this is a gentle way of releasing it. See chapter 5 on page 57 for more information about breathing.

Stand with a roller or half roller across the middle of your back and lean onto it against a wall.

Just rest there, using the weight of your body to allow your tissues to melt around the roller, until you feel a softening.

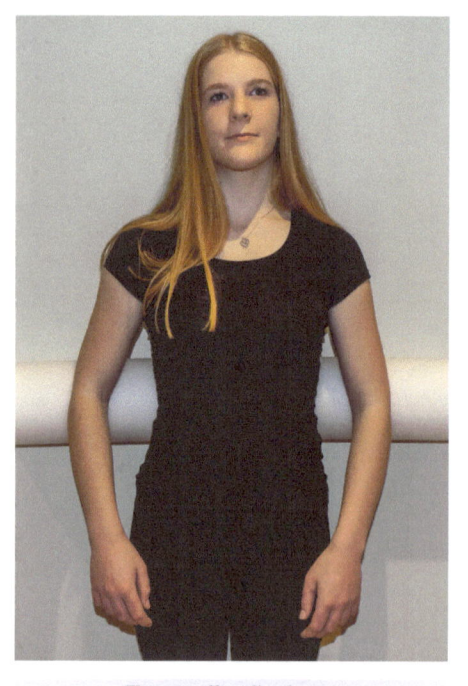

*Foam roller diaphram*

To increase the intensity, try raising your arms above your head. But remember that you are feeling for resistance, not pain. Aim to hold for at least five minutes. This can also be carried out while you are sitting. You can try lying on your back with the foam roller on the floor or bed, but this can be too big a stretch for some people, so go slowly.

## How to help your lower back

### Back release using a ball

This technique focuses on your psoas muscles, which run from the front of your hips on either side, through your pelvis and then attach into the front of your spine, nearly to the level of your diaphragm.

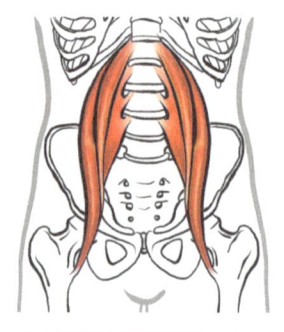

*Psoas muscles*

The best way to access them is from the front. You can find out more about these very important muscles in chapter 3 on page 27.

Lie on your stomach on the floor. On your loosest side locate the bone at the front of your pelvis. Place the tennis ball up from the bone and towards your belly button. Lie face down on the ball for 10 minutes, or as long as is comfortable. Repeat on the tighter side.

Do not do this release if you are pregnant, think you might be pregnant, or have recently had abdominal surgery.

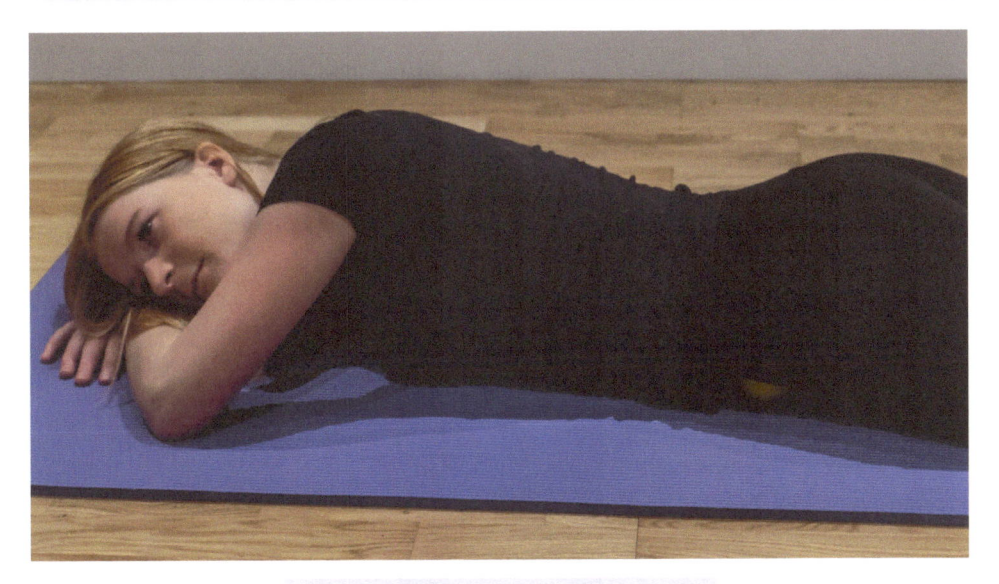

*Ball in psoas muscles*

## Back release in standing

This release is easy to do when you are out and about. It allows you to directly soften your psoas muscles, which can go into spasm. Use this if your back is tight and sore when you get up from sitting, or when you straighten up from bending over.

Stand with equal weight through both legs and hook your thumbs in behind the bones at the front of your pelvis. It may feel very tight and tender there, so just sink in as far as you can comfortably go.

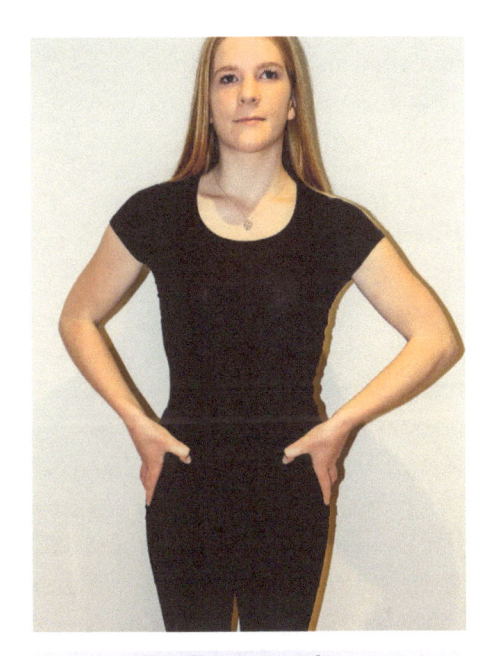

*Standing psoas release*

Then wait for the tightness to start releasing after about two minutes. This will happen gradually, allowing your bottom to tuck in and your back to straighten up. Don't worry if each side releases at different times, just keep the gentle pressure on with both thumbs and wait for them to level up.

It is also good to do when you are still sitting if you feel that your back is beginning to seize up. If you are sitting, it might be a bit harder to find the bones, but the technique is just the same as when you are standing. If you know that your back tends to tense up when you are sitting, practising finding the right place when you are sitting in a chair might be helpful. This allows you to release the tension before you stand up.

### Back release using a foam roller

This is a lovely gentle way to release your whole back and it is great for getting you used to feeling what your body needs.

For the best results, this should be done regularly, and you should aim to spend 20 to 30 minutes on it each time. If you feel this exercise is making any symptoms worse, stop and inform your therapist at your next treatment.

Please note that your body's requirements will be different every time you use your roller. Therefore, remember to follow your body. It doesn't matter how far you move into a position, as long as you stop at the barriers when you feel them.

Choose an area of floor with enough space for you to lie with your arms and legs spread out and place the roller on the floor in the middle.

Sit on the edge of the roller and lower yourself down so your spine is along the length of it, with your head well supported. Keep your knees bent and your feet flat on the floor. Allow your arms to rest on the floor. Remain in this position until your body feels relaxed and completely comfortable. This may take the whole session – if this is the case, do not push your body further.

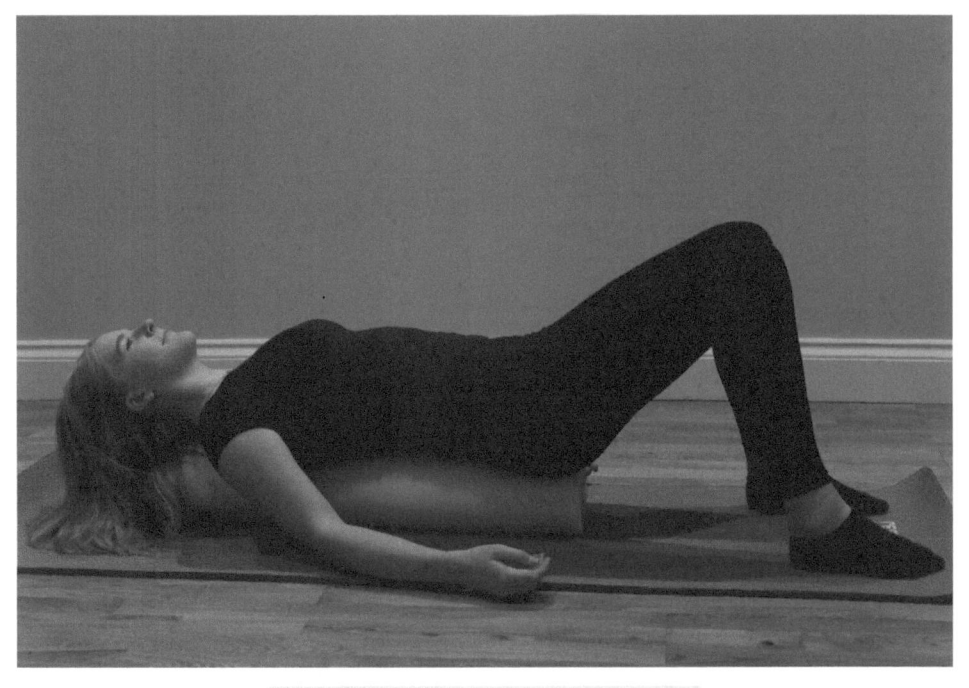

*Spine release with foam roller*

If you feel able, slowly take your arms out to the side, keeping contact with the floor. Stop as soon as you feel pulling and before you feel pain. Remember you may feel things anywhere in your body and your arms might need to be at different levels or heights.
Wait in the position that you feel the tightness until it releases. This will probably take a few minutes.

Do the same with your legs, but one at a time (otherwise you might fall off the roller!). Find a position of tightness and wait for the release.

## The Constructive Rest Position

This is a yoga pose that focuses on allowing your lower back and particularly the psoas muscles to relax. It is a neutral position that reduces muscle tension and can even clear your mind. It is helpful if you have fibromyalgia because of the link between the psoas muscles and your autonomic nervous system, which can affect energy levels and sensitivity to pain.

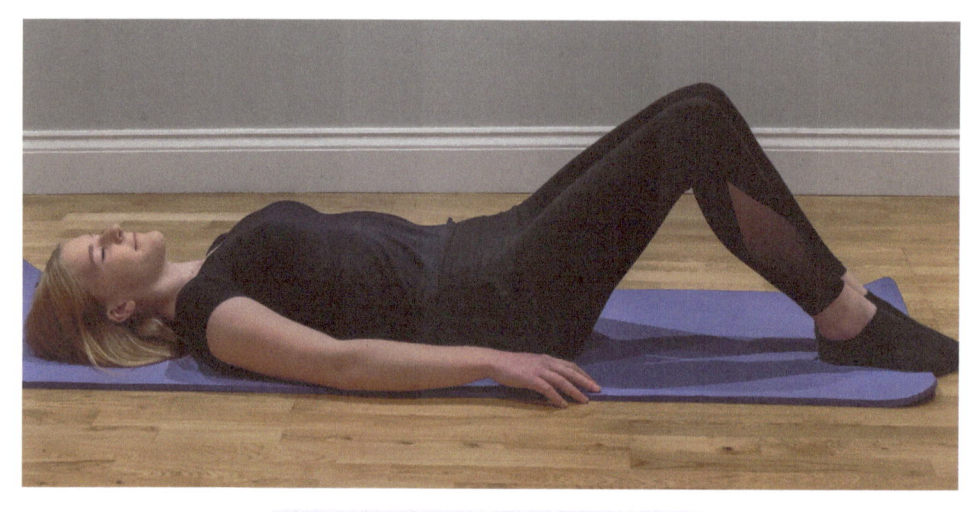

*Constructive rest position*

Lie on your back with your knees bent and your feet on the ground. Your feet should be in line with your sitting bones and far enough away from each other to allow your knees to rest against each other.

You may need a small pillow or towel under your head to support your neck. You can also have your legs raised and resting on a chair or pillows if that is more comfortable for you. Your arms can rest on the floor or on your tummy, whichever you find most relaxing.

Then do nothing.

Focus on your breathing: 4 counts in, pause, 6 counts out. This will help your whole body to relax and let go. Do this for 10-20 minutes a day if you can, remembering to follow your body and build up slowly if you need to. If you have time, longer sessions are advisable or even twice a day.

## How to help your legs

### Releasing the front of your upper leg using a ball

This release focuses on the quadriceps (thigh muscles) and it is very helpful when traditional quad stretches aren't reaching your tightness.

Facing a wall, place the ball at the front of your thigh, just below your hip. Then lean into the wall so that you feel gentle pressure from the ball, but no pain. Wait in that position until you feel your muscle soften, then move the ball down to the next tight area and repeat.

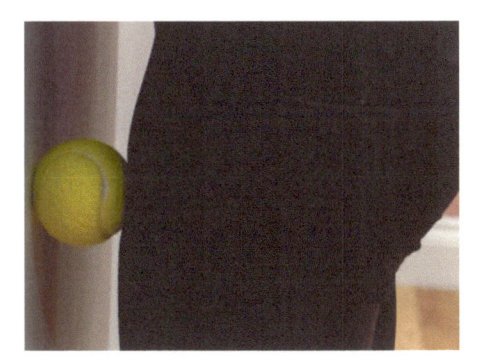

*Ball in thigh*

This release can also be done using a foam roller against the wall or lying on your front on the floor with the ball or roller under your thigh.

## Releasing the back of your upper leg

This release for your hamstrings is a gentler alternative to the traditional stretch.

Lean forward and rest your upper body on the back of a chair or table. Lift your tailbone towards the ceiling and drop your lower back towards the floor, feeling for the release in the back of your legs.

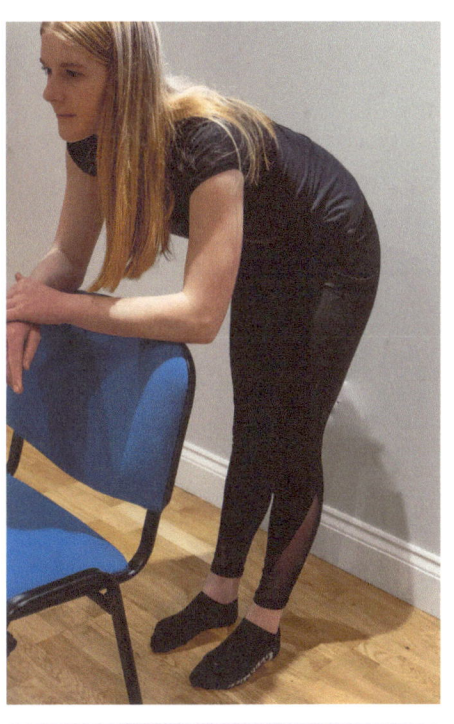

*Hamstrings release*

As your muscles release, allow your body to shift forward, back or to either side to access the next layer of restriction. Actively lower your back further towards the floor, while lifting your tailbone higher to increase elongation. Try with both legs together or one leg at a time, with your non-weight bearing foot resting on top of the weight bearing foot.

## Releasing the backs of your upper legs with a foam roller.

This is a lovely gentle way of softening down the backs of both your legs. To start with, you will probably need to release the whole of the muscles, but as you progress, you will be able to feel which areas need more attention.

Sit or lie with your legs straight and your back supported. Place the foam roller across the back of both your legs, just below your buttocks. Allow your legs to rest onto the roller and wait until you feel the muscles soften. Then move the roller down your legs to the next tight area. You can continue down your legs in this way to release your calves too.

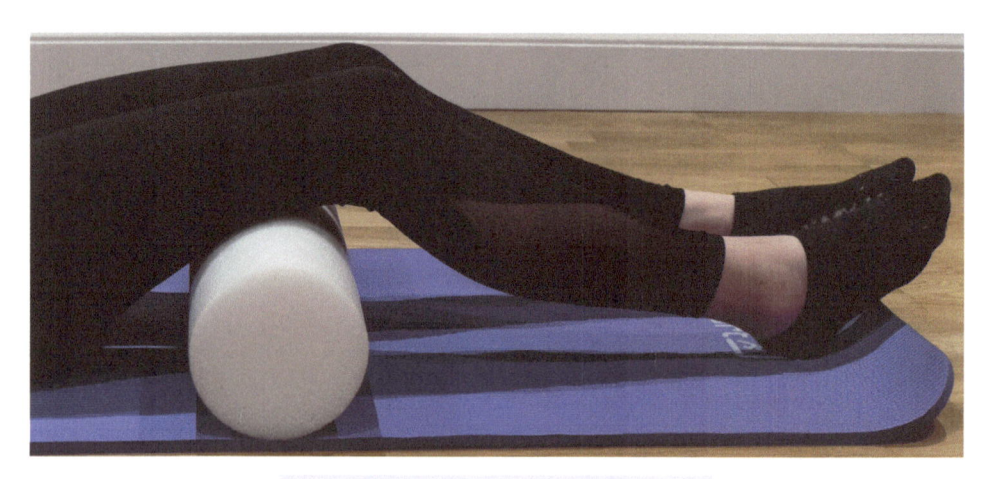

*Foam roller to backs of legs*

## Releasing the tendon on the outside of your upper leg with a foam roller

This tendon is called the iliotibial (or IT) band and it often gets very tight and tender, especially in athletes. This way of using the foam roller to release it should be pain-free, so it is a great alternative to lying on the roller.

Place a foam roller horizontally against a wall, just below your hip height. Stand side-on to a wall and rest the outside of your upper leg against the roller. Lean onto the roller with just enough weight that you can feel a gentle pressure but no pain.

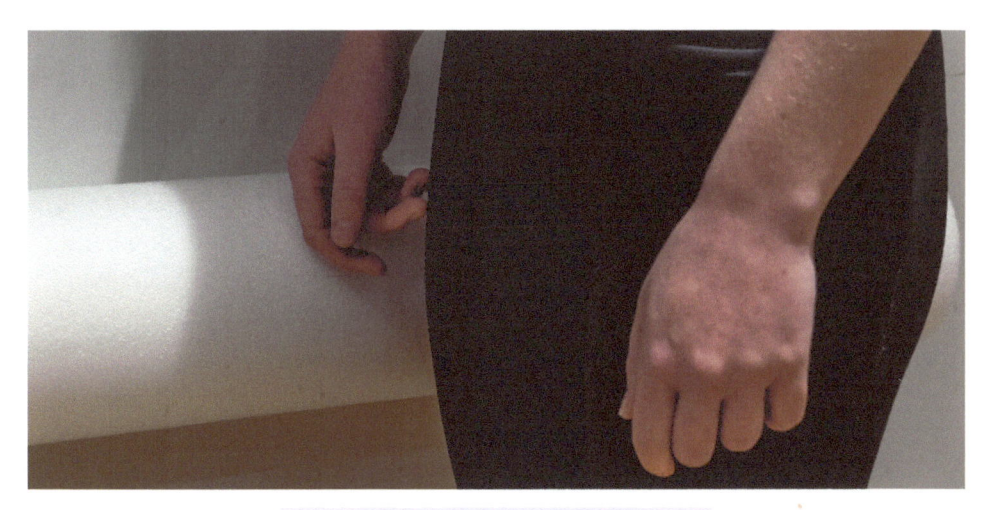

*Foam roller to side of legs*

Wait until you feel your leg softening, then shift the roller down your leg to the next tight point and repeat. This can be done all the way down to your knee. You can also start at your knee and work up if you find that way round works better for you. Check your other leg, as the IT band is usually tight on both sides.

## Seated contract / relax exercise to release your hips

If you find it difficult to open your hips out – for instance, when getting in and out of a car – this technique can help.

Sit on a firm chair with both feet flat on the floor and slightly apart to start with. Make a fist with both hands and place them on the inside of your knees so they are touching each other. You could use a round football instead if you find it easier.

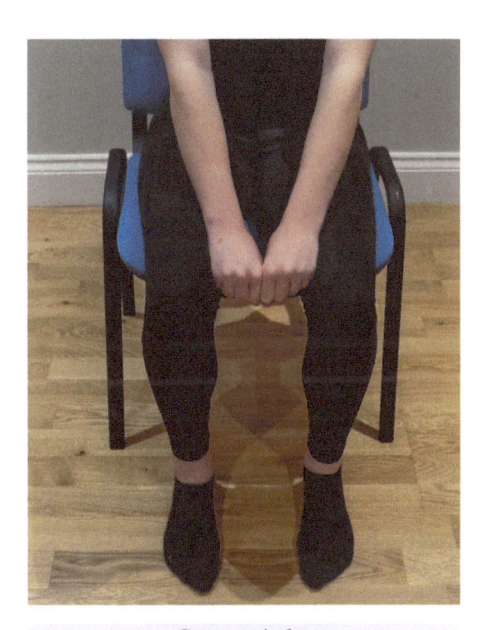

*Contract/relax*

Squeeze both knees in towards each other as tightly as you can so that you are squashing your fists or the ball. Hold this strong contraction for a count of five, then very slowly soften your legs and release the grip until both legs are fully relaxed. Repeat three times.

**Buttocks release**

This focuses on your piriformis muscle, which lies under the gluteus maximus muscle (buttock cheek). It can be very painful when it gets tight. This is a good way of releasing it but remember to go slowly and check both sides.

Lie on your back with the leg on your good side straight and bend the opposite knee up. Place the foot of your bent leg flat on the surface on the outside of your straight knee. Lower your bent knee towards the inside of your body and increase the stretch by moving your knee further diagonally with the opposite hand. Hold the position until you feel the release in your buttock (usually 3-5 minutes).

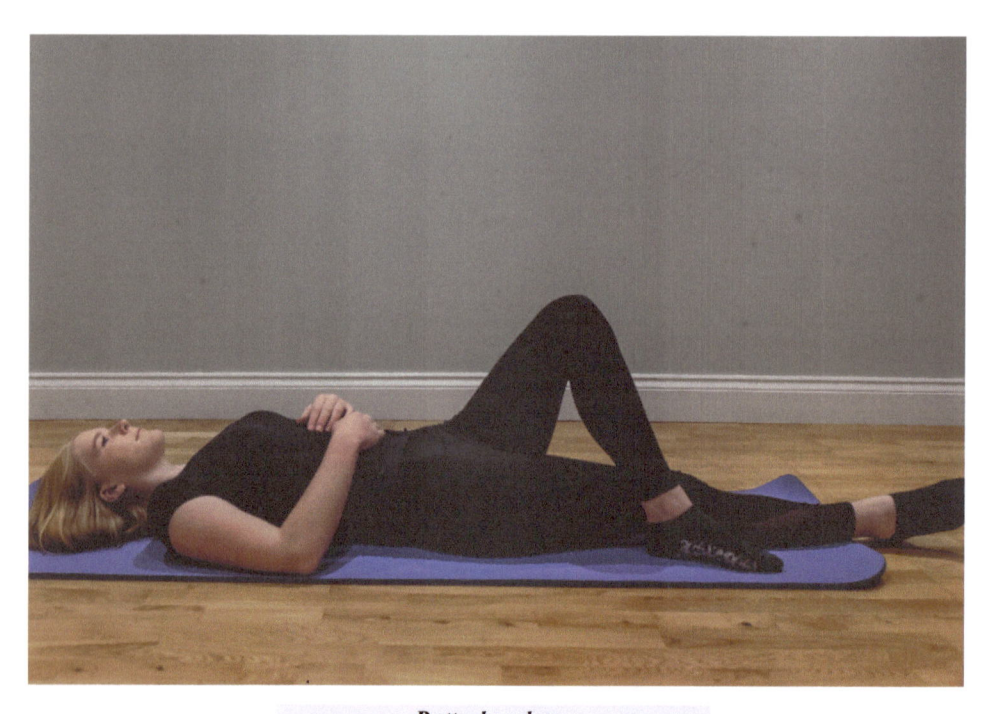

*Buttocks release*

## Calf release using a ball

If you have a point of tension and tenderness in your calf that doesn't release with stretching, this can really help. Don't focus on the pain though – try to feel for tension. If you do find a painful area, move the ball slightly to the side of it.

Sitting on the floor or lying on a mat, place a tennis ball under the tight part of your calf. Allow the tissue to sink over the ball and wait for 3-5 minutes until you feel a release. Move the ball to further tight spots on your calf and repeat as above. Repeat on the other leg. This exercise can also be completed seated whilst leaning against a wall.

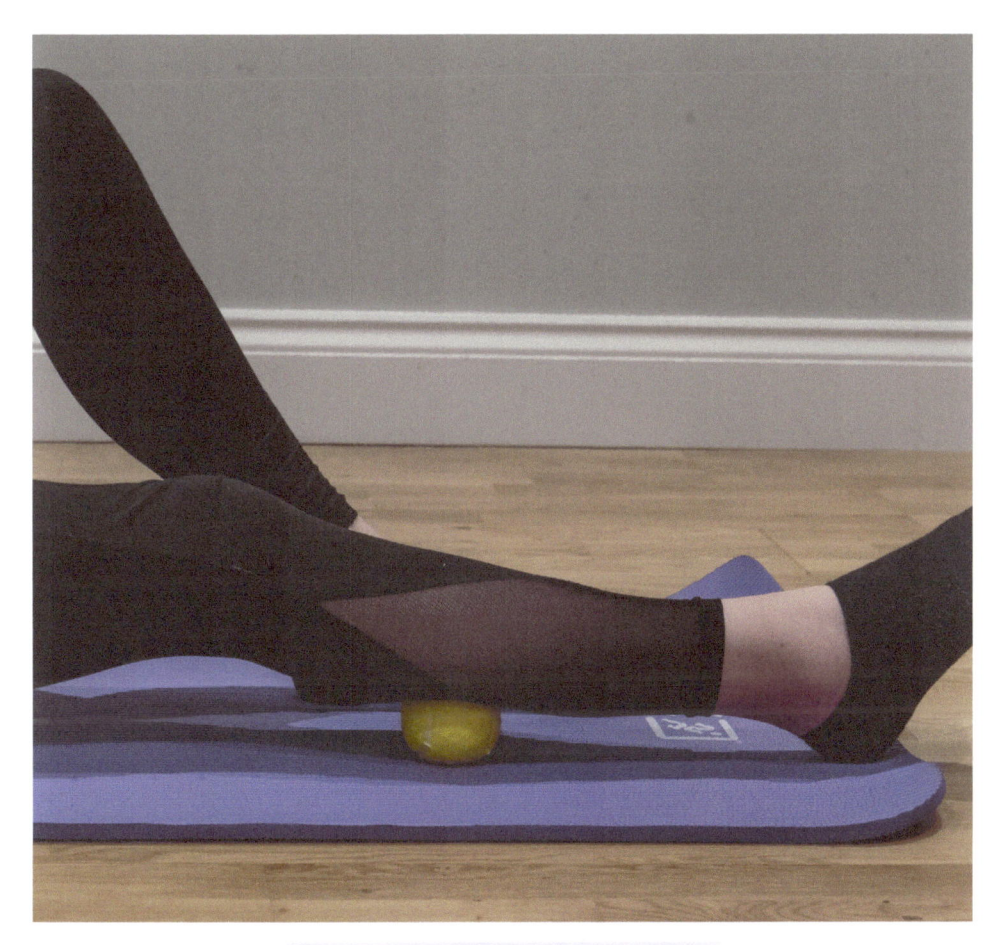

*Ball in calf*

## For tired legs

Lying with your legs leaning up against the wall is so relaxing and is great to relieve tired, achy legs at the end of a hard day.

Lie on your back with your hips as close to a wall as possible and your legs up against the wall. Bring your legs slightly apart and roll your feet down towards you to lengthen the outside of your feet and calves. You can then open your legs out along the wall to release your inner thighs. Remember, never stretch into pain, but find a tight point and wait there until it releases. This can be done on the floor or a bed.

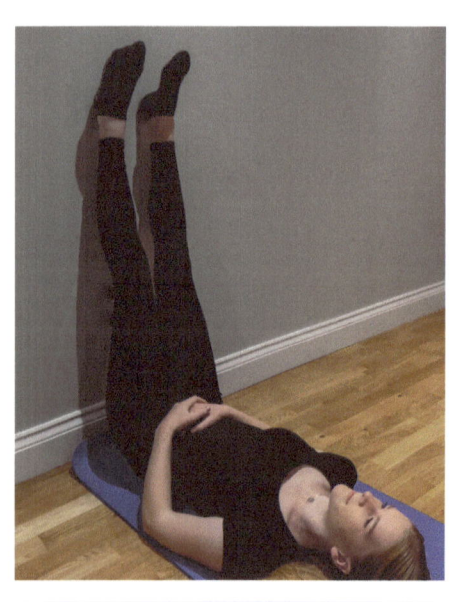

*Legs up the wall*

## How to help your arms

### Elbow release

This can be used to relieve the symptoms of tennis and golfer's elbow as well as after injury. Remember to go slowly and gently.

Straighten your arm out in front of you as far as is comfortable, with your palm facing downwards. Let your wrist relax so your hand drops down and then use your other hand to very gently increase the stretch until you feel a pull into your forearm.
Do not stretch into pain.

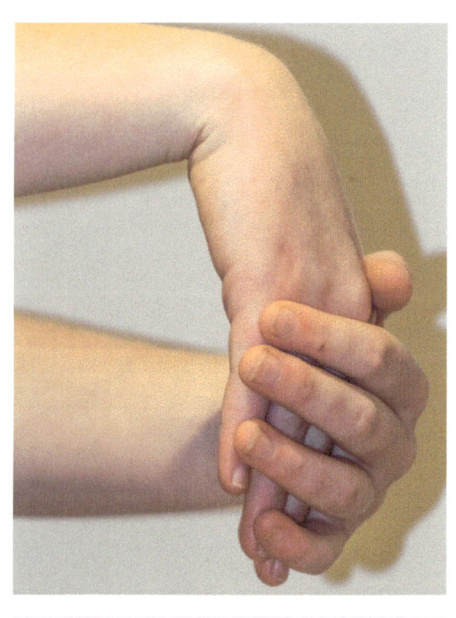

*Wrist down*

Hold that gentle pull until you feel it soften and ease up then bring your hand back to neutral. Next, keeping your arm straight, bend your wrist up so your hand moves towards the ceiling and hold at the point that you feel a gentle pull, until it releases.

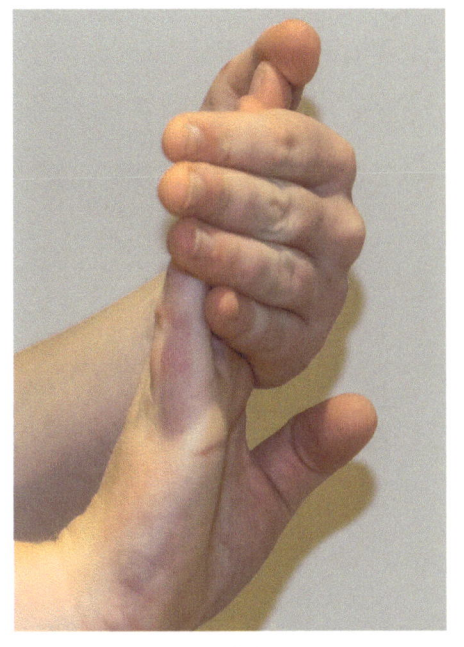

*Wrist up*

## Shoulder release

This is a good way of starting to get your shoulder moving again if it is very stiff and sore, such as after rotator cuff injury and inflammation or frozen shoulder (see chapter 4 on page 35 for more information).

Cradle the elbow on your sore side in your opposite hand, completely relaxing your arm. Using your good arm and starting small, take your elbow round in gradually increasing circles. Do not push into painful areas, but if you feel resistance and the feeling that it will become painful if you keep going, rest at that point.

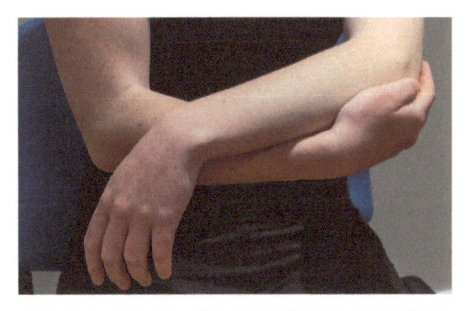

*Shoulder release*

Keep your elbow relaxed into your hand until you feel it soften. Then you can repeat and find other points of tension.

## Chest release

Choose this release to improve your posture if you have rounded shoulders, to improve your breathing capacity and to open up your shoulder joint.

The door frame stretch a great release that can be done anywhere that has a door.
Remember, never force or move into pain, just feel for your comfortable end point and wait there until the area softens.

This release should be done on both sides, and if one side is worse than the other, do the best side first. This is to make things easier for your body to change, and by releasing the looser side you will start to open up the tighter side before you get there.

Stand in the doorway with the side you are working on next to the door frame. With your elbow bent and relaxed, place the palm of your hand facing forwards, flat onto the door frame.

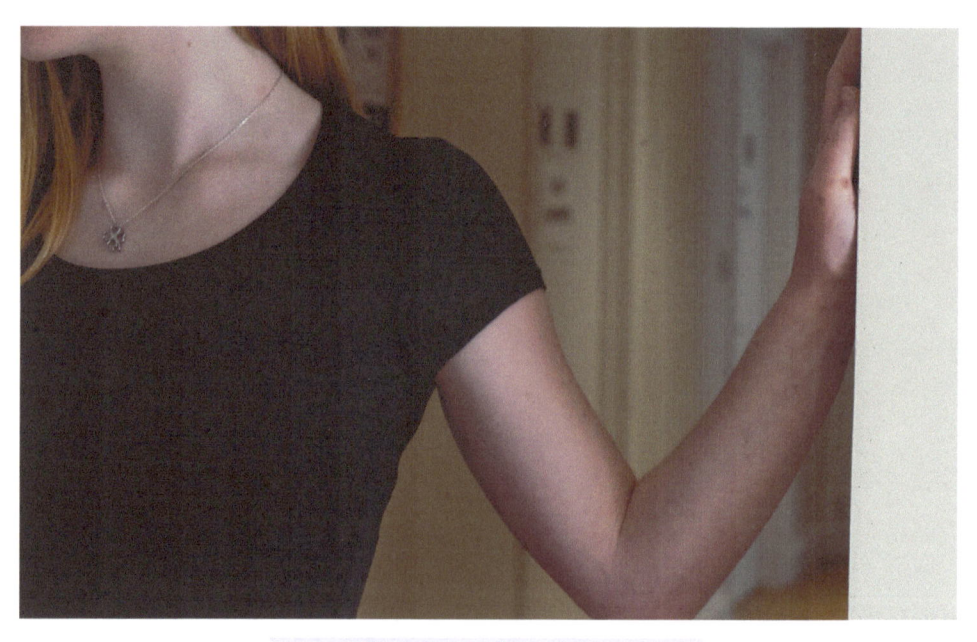

*Door frame chest release*

Slowly lean into the doorway until you feel a gentle pull in the front of your shoulder and into your chest. Then wait at that point until you feel that the pull has lessened or that you are able to move further into the doorway with your body. You can then slowly bring your body back to the centre and relax your arm, or wait at the next pull that you feel, and repeat.

## Shoulder blade release

The door frame lean is good for releasing around your shoulder blade and it can improve your posture if one of your shoulders sits further forward than the other. The shoulder that is being held further back will develop more tension, which will cause a twist through your trunk.

This release can also be done with the corner of a wall or post, but I find that door frames work best for me.

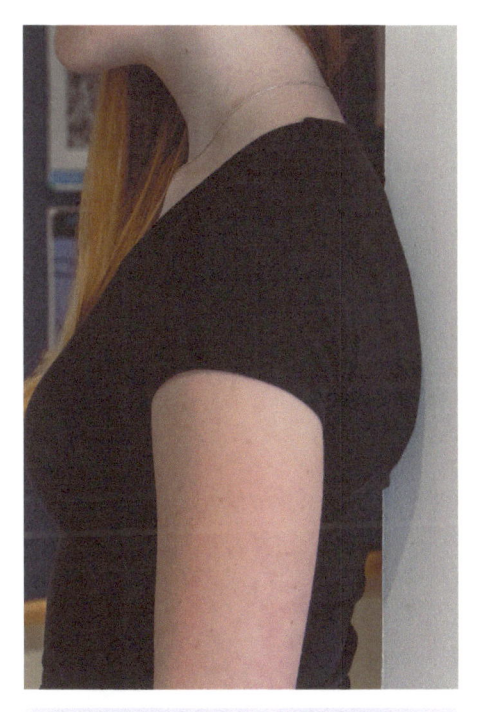

*Door frame shoulder blade release*

Stand with the inside of your shoulder blade against the corner of the door jamb and gently lean into it, using your body weight, not force. Stop before it is painful, waiting wherever you feel resistance. As your tension starts to release, slowly allow yourself to sink further onto the corner of the door frame. Wait until you feel that the shoulder on that side is able to fall forwards slightly or that the arm drops further as the tension releases.

## How to help your hands and feet

### Releasing your hand using a ball

Use this technique if your hands get stiff and sore after using them, if you have arthritic fingers, or after injury.

Sit in a comfortable position with your shoulders relaxed. Rest your hand over the top of a tennis ball or one of similar size, on a flat surface. Gently start to roll the ball under your hand but keep your fingers relaxed – they shouldn't be gripping the ball at all. If you feel that the rolling movement slows or stops, rest and wait in that position, allowing the weight of your hand to sink onto the ball.

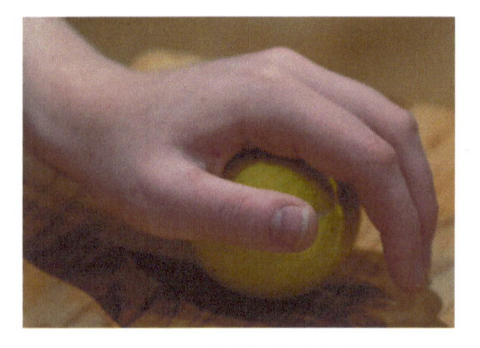

*Hand on ball*

Once the restriction softens and releases, you will easily be able to roll on the ball again until the next stop. It may take a few minutes for the tightness to release but it is worth being patient and waiting for it to change properly.

The idea of this exercise is to feel and find the tight bits, which will be in different places each time you do it. Never push into pain – if a spot is very tender, just roll off it slightly so that you can release the tissue around the painful area.

## Finger pulls

This is a great way for you to treat yourself and it can be done anywhere. Each of your fingers has three joints which can all be affected by pain and stiffness. By gently releasing the soft tissues around the joints, you will increase the blood flow to the area and take the strain of the joint. You can do this for all your fingers if you find that both your hands tighten up, if you are gripping for a long time, or working in the cold. Or if you only have one or two affected fingers, it is fine to just do the self-treatment on them.

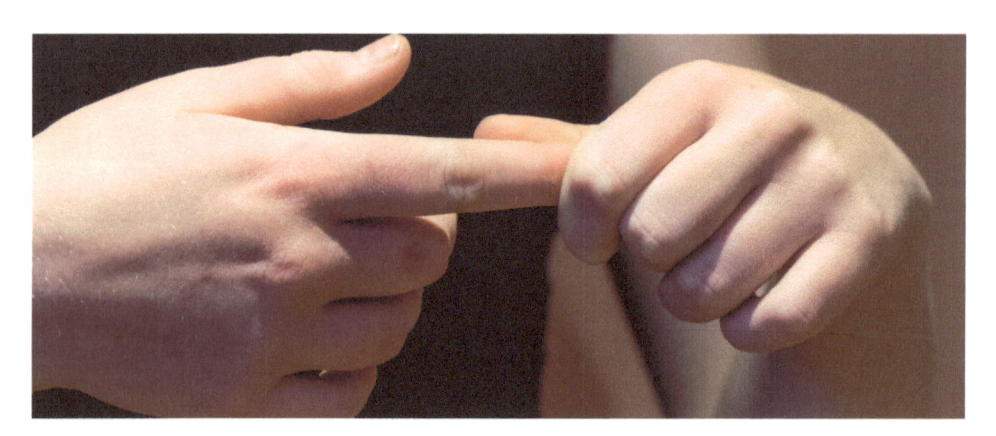

*Finger pulls*

Rest your arm in a comfortable position, then gently hold the finger that you are going to treat between the thumb and first finger of your other hand. Very slowly start to apply a gentle traction to pull your finger, without moving over the skin. It is very important to stay focussed so that you can feel as soon as you feel a resistance to the pull. Never pull into pain. Once you have found the tightness, maintain the traction until you feel your finger soften or lengthen. Then slowly release your pull and move on to the next finger as needed.

## Release for the tops of your feet

If your feet feel uncomfortable in the kneeling position or after they have been in the same position for a while, this can help.

Sitting on a chair, bend your knees and draw your feet back to allow your toes to tuck underneath you and rest on floor. Hold the position for 3-5 minutes. You will feel releases in the tops of your feet and shins. This exercise could be done while working at a desk or on a computer. You can choose to do one leg at a time or both together.

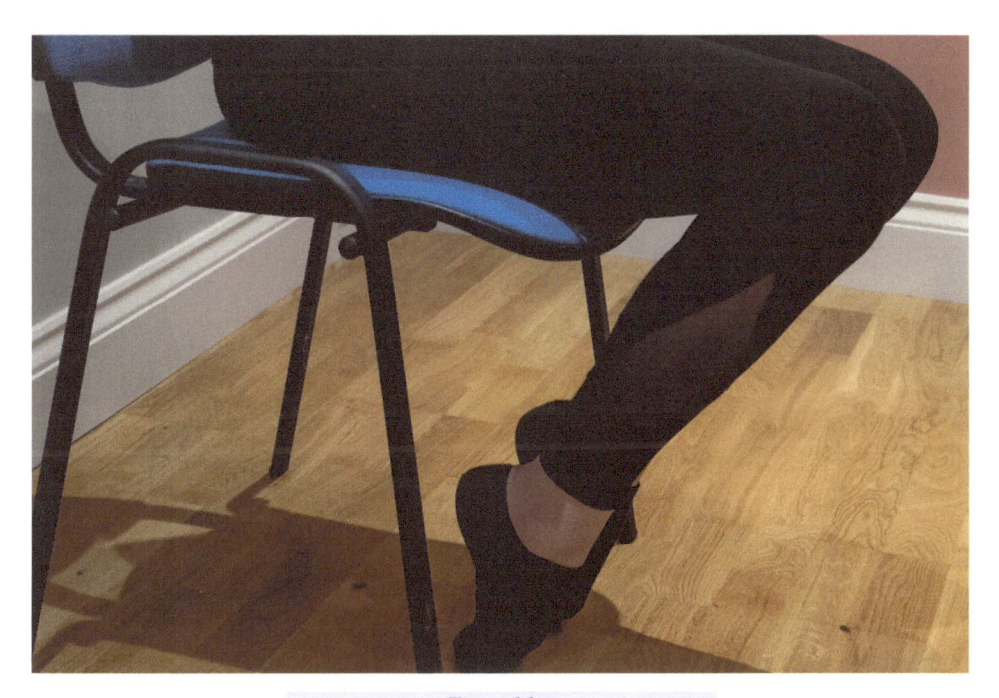

*Tops of feet*

## Releasing your foot on a ball

This is great for plantar fasciitis and arthritic joints in your feet.

Sit with the sole of your affected foot resting onto a small ball. Some people use golf balls or spiky Pilates balls, which is fine if it works for you, but please go gently as too much pressure can cause bruising.

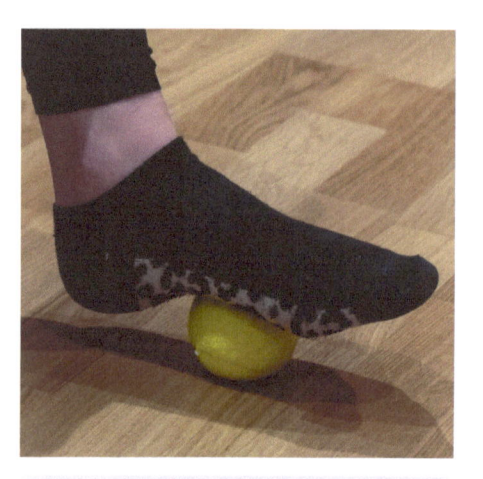

*Foot on ball*

Slowly roll your foot over the ball for a couple of minutes. If you find a spot that is very tight, just rest in that position until you feel it change and release. If any points are too painful to apply pressure into, then don't – you will still be helping those areas if you work around them.

## Foot on foot release

Sit with your affected foot on the floor and your knee bent at right-angles. Place your other foot on the top of the affected foot in whatever position feels right.

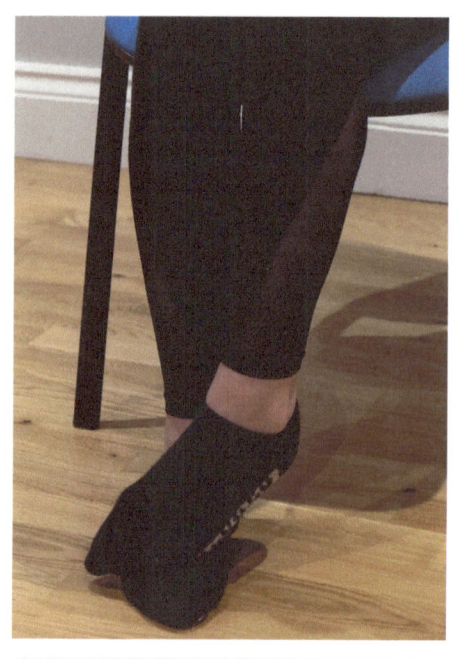

*Foot on foot*

Apply gentle pressure from your top foot and hold for at least five minutes. If you feel that you need extra pressure, you can also push down through the knee of the affected foot. But remember that you are not looking for pain, just your barrier. Then, wait and sink down as your foot opens up. Stop if you have any increase in pain.

## How to help your head and face

### Releasing your temples

These points either side of your forehead often hold tension that can lead to jaw problems and stress headaches.

Sit with your back and shoulders relaxed. Using both hands, place your fingertips on each side of your head, resting on your temples. Gently test the movement by moving your fingers up and down and backwards and forwards (without sliding on the skin), to find the areas of resistance. These are likely to be different on each side. Hold in this position until you feel a release. This may take 3-5 minutes. As you feel the releases, you can follow to the next area of resistance and repeat the process.

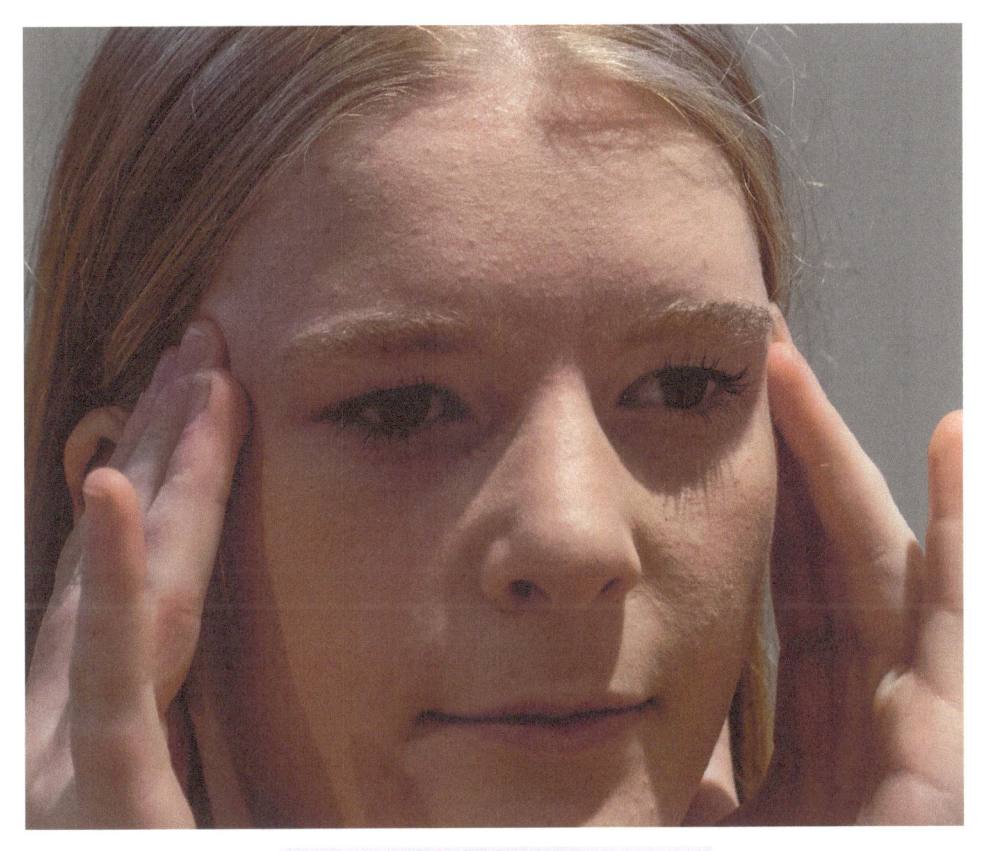

*Treating temples*

## Releasing your forehead

Tension held here can cause headaches and eye strain, so this easy release should be done as soon as you become aware of your forehead tightening up.

Sit with your back and shoulders relaxed. Place the fingertips of both hands onto your forehead and allow them to sink in. Gently test the movement by moving your fingers up and down and backwards and forwards (without sliding on the skin), to find the areas of resistance. Hold in this position until you feel a release. This may take 3-5 minutes. As it releases, you can follow to the next area of resistance and repeat the process.

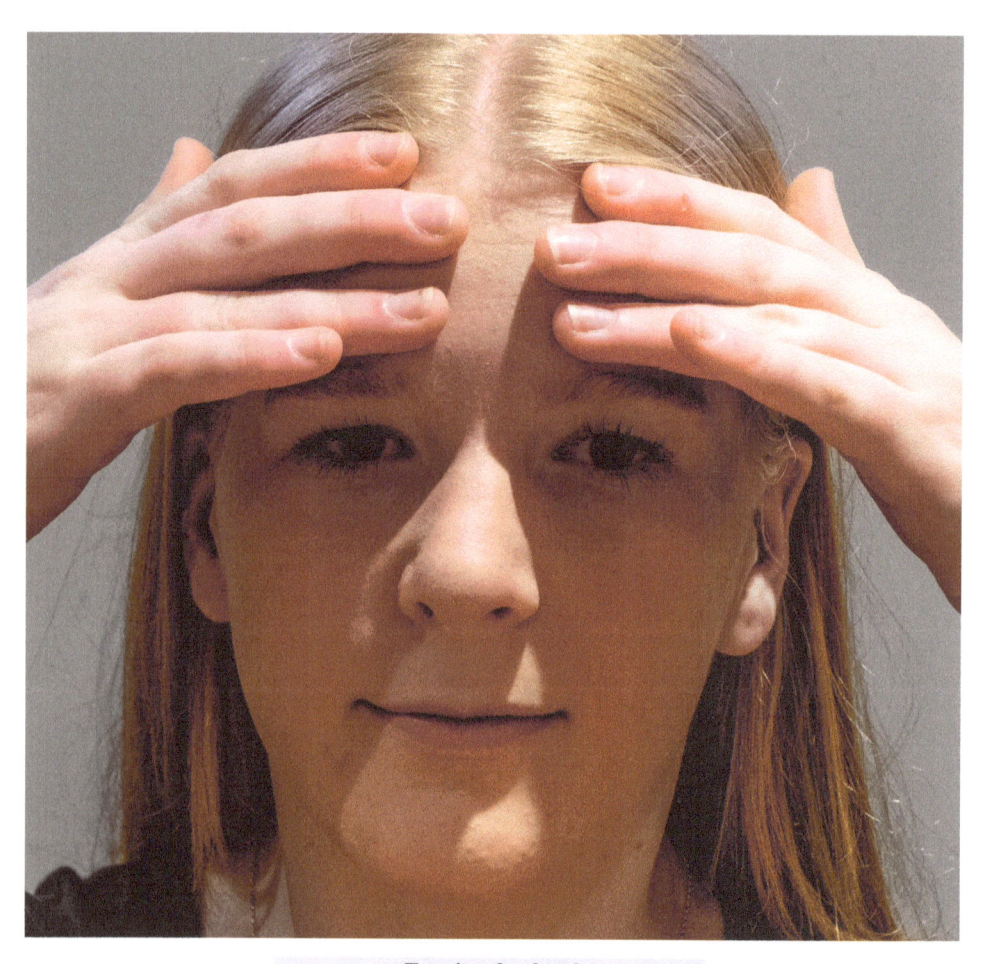

*Treating forehead*

## Sinus release

Blocked sinuses are so uncomfortable, and this is a gentle way of encouraging them to drain.

Sit with your elbows bent and supported and place the fingertips of both your hands under your cheek bones. Allow your fingers to sink in and hold in this position until you feel a release. This may take 3-5 minutes. As you feel the releases, you can follow to the next area of resistance and repeat the process.

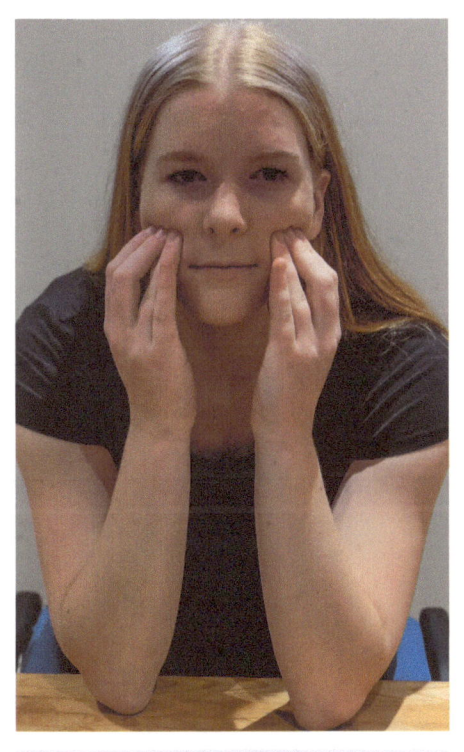

*Treating sinuses*

## Hair pull

Using your hair as a way of relieving tension in your head allows you to access deep areas that are hard to reach. You can release any area of your head, not just the temples.

Sitting or lying, gently take hold of a handful of hair on each temple. Keeping your shoulders relaxed, pull the hair out to the sides and backwards until you feel a resistance. Hold in this position until you feel a release. This may take three to five minutes. As your tension releases, you can follow to the next area of resistance and repeat the process.

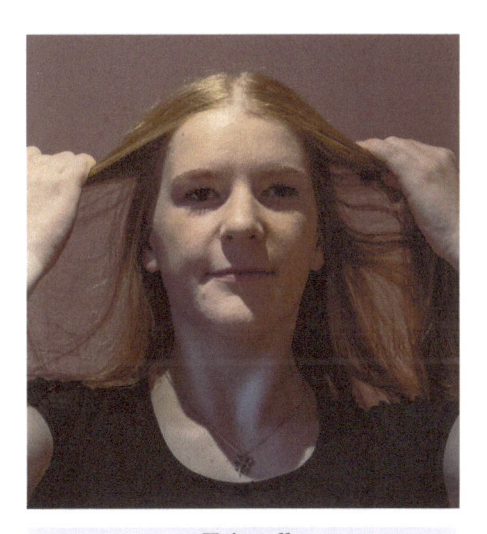

*Hair pull*

## Ear pulls

This is a great way of clearing blocked ears when you are flying, and after a cold or infection.

Take hold of your ear, holding the cartilage either side with your thumb and 1st finger.
Gently pull outwards (away from your head) and backwards until you feel resistance. Hold the position for 3 – 5 minutes until you feel a release. As you feel the release, increase the pull, and when you feel more resistance, wait again. Repeat on the other ear.

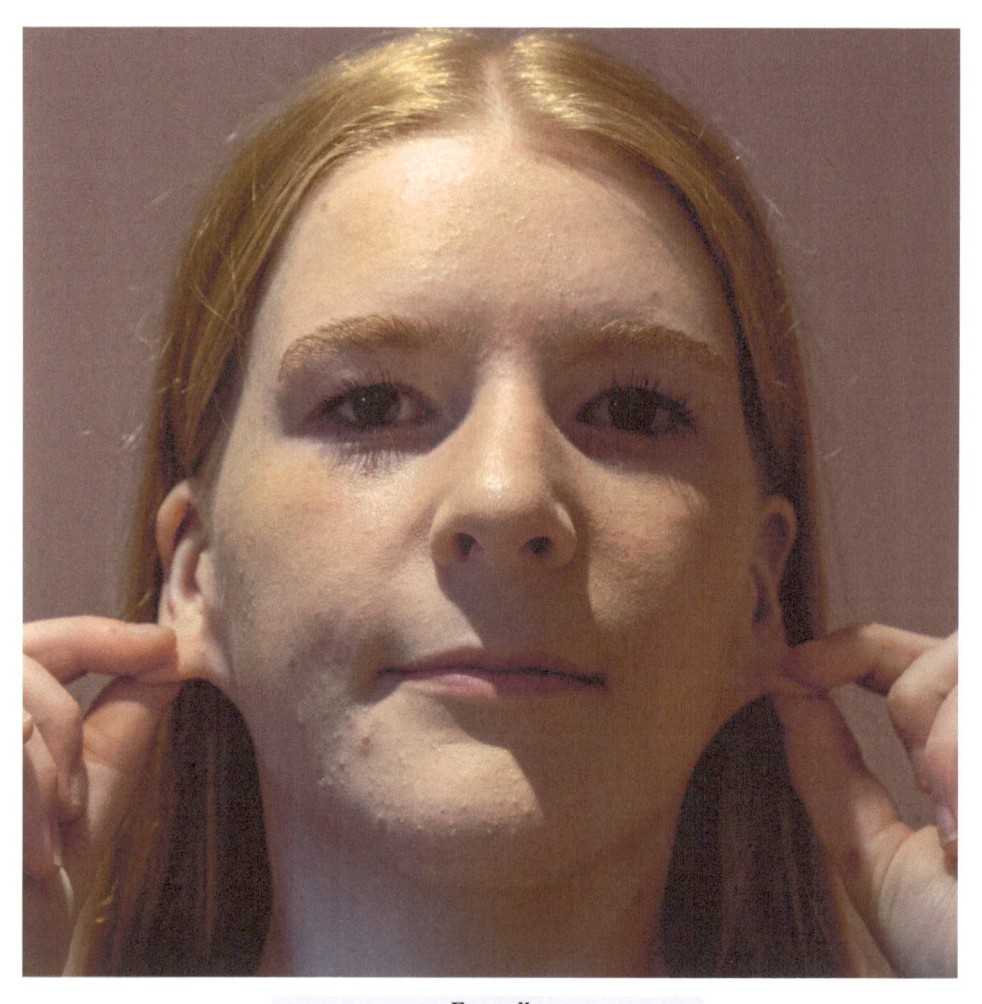

*Ear pull*

# References

1. K. R. Meltzer, T. V. Cao, J. F. Schad, H. King, S. T. Stoll, and P. R. Standley. *"In Vitro Modeling of Repetitive Motion Injury and Myofascial Release."* Journal of Bodywork and Movement Therapies 14, no. 2 (2010): 162–71.

2. Meltzer KR, Standley PR. Modelled repetitive motion strain and indirect osteopathic manipulation techniques in regulation of human fibroblast proliferation and interleukin secretion." J Am Osteopath Assoc. 2007;107(12):527-536

3. C. Beardsley and J. Skarabot. *"Effects of Self-Myofascial Release: A Systemic Review"* Journal of Bodywork and Movement Therapies 19, no 4 (2015): 747-58

4. P.F. Curran, R.D. Fiore, and J.J. Crisco. *"A Comparison of the Pressure Exerted on Soft Tissue by 2 Myofascial Rollers."* Journal of Sport Rehabilitation 17, no 4 (2008):432-42.

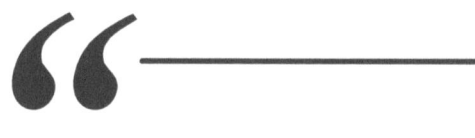

> *Give yourself permission to let go.*
>
> John F. Barnes

# CHAPTER 8

# MYOFASCIAL RELEASE

## What is myofascial release?

Developed by physiotherapist John F. Barnes, myofascial release (MFR) is a safe, gentle, hands-on treatment that works with your body to untangle the restrictions that cause pain, tension and inflammation. He defines it as an 'innovative and highly effective whole-body approach for the evaluation and treatment of pain and dysfunction.'[1]

As discussed in chapter 1 on page 7, your fascial system connects every cell in your body via a continuous web of connective tissue, with the gloopy ground substance lying in-between. The ground substance reacts to physical and emotional stress and then becomes more solid, preventing your body from being able to adapt to things and leading to symptoms and illness.

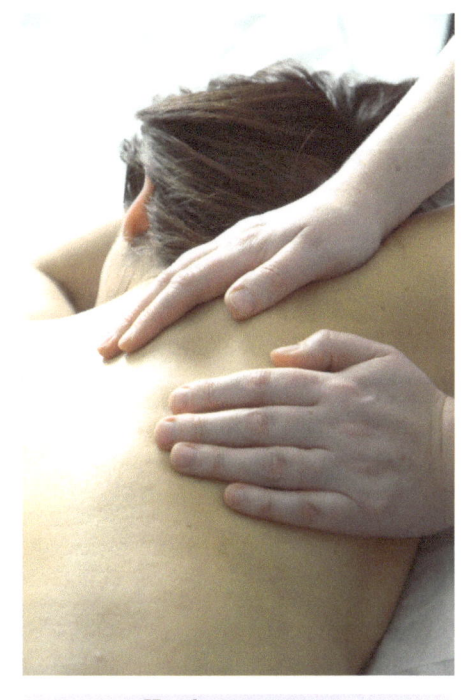

*Hands-on treatment*

It is thixotropic, meaning that it becomes more fluid after 90 to 120 seconds of warmth and gentle, sustained pressure.[2] Once the pressure is taken off the connective tissue fibres, they are able to start to release and gradually come back to their optimum position. This is why using a hot pack or having a warm bath feel so relaxing and can help to reduce pain and stiffness.

During treatment this thixotropic reaction is initiated from the therapist's hands. They are able to use this reaction to feel where the restrictions are coming from and to gently follow and release them. As myofascial release treatment never forces the patient's body, it is very safe and enables the therapist to truly follow what they need, getting long-term results. It also allows them to work very deeply without pain, so most patients find it a very relaxing experience.

This property is similar to that found in Blu Tack; when it is cold and hasn't been used for a long time, is it hard and ungiving. As you work it with your fingers, applying warmth and pressure, it gradually becomes more elastic and stretchier.

By sinking down to the patient's barrier (as far as the tissue will give without forcing it), the therapist waits for the myofascia to start to soften and let go. With training and experience, myofascial release therapists can follow the releases that occur and also feel other areas of restriction in the body that are related.

In this way, we are able to feel our way through your tissues, releasing and then stretching until the next restriction. As many symptoms begin in response to irritation from tightness in the myofascia elsewhere in the body, it is usual for treatment to begin in a different part of the body to where the problem is felt.

Rather like unpicking a ball of string that is full of knots, it is important to release your body in the right order. The therapist can feel where the next knot along is in your body, and just like the next knot in the ball of string, this may be on the other side of your body.

Some patients are very aware of the changes that occur during myofascial release treatment and are able to feel where in their body the therapist needs to work next. Others only feel the movement under the therapist's hands. Whether or not you can feel the subtle changes, they are still happening and are potentially altering your whole body via the myofascial network.

Restrictions and scar tissue can cause many symptoms that are not traditionally treated by body work. Myofascial release works with your body to open these up. It is very effective for problems that have been there for years, as well as acute injuries.

## What does it involve?

The exact structure of the treatment will vary from therapist to therapist, but to give you an idea of what to expect if you decide to go for myofascial release treatment, I am going to describe what happens in my Treatment Centre.

### Assessment

We start off with a video phone call, during which we will ask you about your past medical history and about the symptoms you are currently experiencing. We will also explain about the treatment and answer any questions that you may have.

Your past medical history is very relevant, as everything from how you were born onwards has the potential to cause your fascial system to tighten up. Even relatively minor events and things that you may not have a memory of will be affecting your body today and could be contributing to your current symptoms.

Following your initial consultation, your first session will include a further short assessment, and we will ask that you sign our consent form prior to hands-on treatment.

We will assess your posture and look at any movements that are restricted by pain or stiffness. It is common for symptoms to occur in a different part of the body to where the problem originates, so treatment may not always be where you are experiencing pain.

Myofascial release is a hands-on treatment that works best on skin, rather than through material. You may therefore be asked to take clothes off down to your underwear, depending on the condition being treated. Some people prefer to bring shorts and a vest top to change into – this is a personal preference. If you think you will struggle to have skin on skin contact, please tell us and we will find a way that works for you.

Once the session is complete, we will discuss your ongoing treatment with you. The number of sessions required varies from patient to patient, even those with the same symptoms, as each person is unique and individual. As a general rule, the longer a symptom has been present, the longer it takes to resolve it. It may be possible to give you an idea of how many sessions you will require, but we cannot tell exactly.

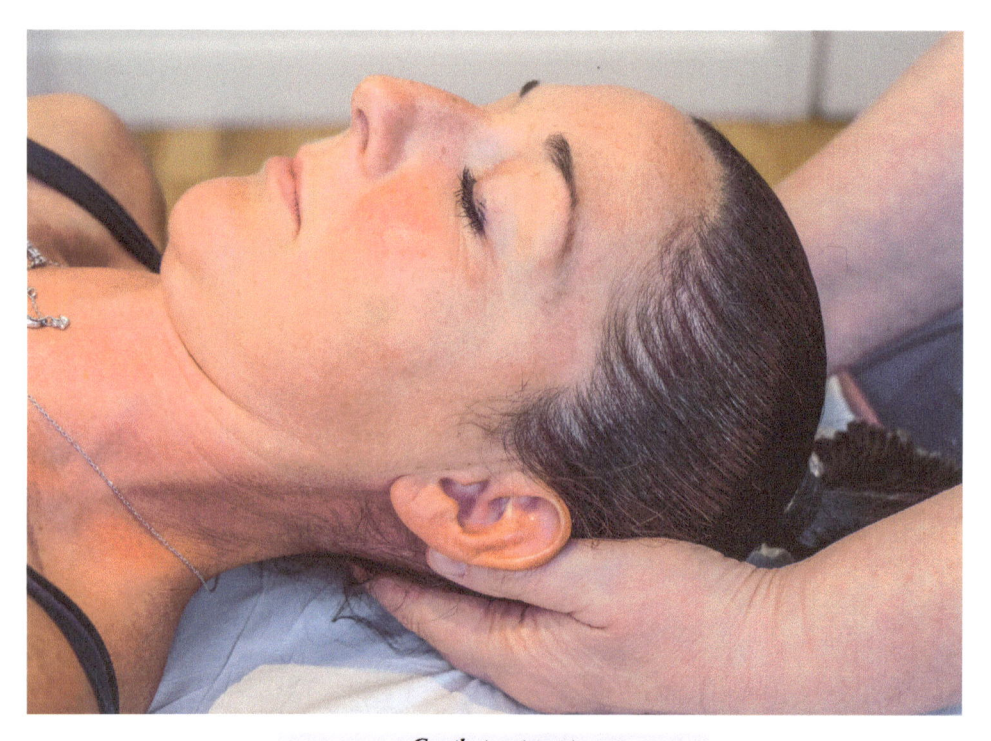

*Gentle treatment*

## Treatment

Some people feel immediate benefits after the treatment, while others find that symptoms change over the next couple of days. Everybody will respond in their own way, and you will start to learn how your body responds as you go through the course of treatment.

It is very important to communicate with us how you feel your treatment is progressing and what your expectations are. Myofascial release is not a 'quick fix', but if you are able to complete the course of treatment that your body needs, it is often possible to get long-lasting results that enable you to manage even chronic conditions yourself.

Throughout your treatment, you are encouraged to tell us what you are feeling. This helps us to follow your body and also helps you to work with your body day to day. It is also important to tell your therapist immediately if you want them to stop whatever they are doing.

As discussed in chapter 2 on page 15, physical and emotional traumas are connected and are often held together in your tissues. So, it is quite common for you to experience emotional releases during the treatment. These cannot be planned or predicted, and you do not need to know why or what event the emotion was specifically related to. In my experience, when emotions do come up during or after treatment, it is when you are ready to release them and is never harmful.

Please remember to make sure you are well hydrated to get the best out of your treatment. To help you with this, we provide filtered drinking water, and we encourage our patients to bring their own drinking bottles to refill.

**Healing crisis**

Occasionally, following a treatment, symptoms may get worse before they get better. This is a normal response to treatments like this that affect the whole body and is nothing to worry about.

Your body is starting to heal itself, and this process commences with the elimination of toxins. When toxins are filtered into the bloodstream quicker than they can be eliminated, it can make you feel as if your symptoms are worsening. You may also find that previous injuries or conditions feel as if they are flaring up.[3]

It is normal to feel energised, calm, relaxed, exhausted, moody, emotional, or anywhere in between. Try to tune in to your body and follow whatever is coming up — and most of all, be gentle with yourself.

To help alleviate the crisis, you should drink plenty of water to help your body flush out the toxins. You may also feel more tired than usual, so try to rest when you can.

A healing crisis is actually a positive sign; it shows that the treatment is having an effect. If you look after yourself it should pass quickly, usually in 1-3 days. Remember that healing is a process that will take time and that it is normal to experience fluctuations in your symptoms.

Your therapist should be able to advise you on how you can help yourself at home in-between appointments. This may include self-treatment techniques, stretches or exercises similar to those shown in this book.

## Unwinding

Sometimes during your treatment, you may experience movements that feel as though your therapist is initiating them. These are spontaneous movements known as unwinding. Animals and children do this naturally, they stretch and move without conscious thought as their body needs to.

Unwinding is a safe and effective way to release restrictions in the fascia by using the body's natural movements. As the restrictions are released, your body begins to move, gradually self-correcting as the fascia returns to its normal state.[4]

### *What does unwinding feel like?*

- Like you are moving in zero gravity.
- Your body feels lighter.
- You may think your therapist is moving you.
- You may get a tingling sensation.
- Your movements may feel jerky.
- Movements may become faster as the tissue releases.

- You may notice that your body goes into positions that you know you cannot do.

You may also feel that you want to cry, laugh, shout, or generally feel emotional. This is because as the fascia corrects itself, it may release the emotions that were present when the injury or trauma occurred.

Giving yourself permission to experience unwinding, rather than resisting, is extremely beneficial. Because the movement is coming from your body, it can never *"go too far"* and therefore will never strain or injure you.

Myofascial release is different from many other types of therapy in that the releases that start during your treatment continue for hours or even days after you leave. This is because it changes restrictions and holding patterns deep within the connective tissue of the body.

## References

1. J. Barnes. *"Healing Ancient Wounds: The Renegade's Wisdom."* Paoli, PA: Rehabilitation Services. 2000.

2. H. Freundlich. *"Some Recent Work on Gels."* Journal of Physical Chemistry 41, no. 7 (1937): 901 – 10. doi:10.1021/j150385a001.

3. B. Fife *"The Healing Crisis"* Piccadilly Books Ltd 2010

4. J. Barnes in CM Davis *"Integrative Therapies in Rehabilitation"* SLACK Incorporated: 2017

> *Say to yourself, 'I survived'.*

John F. Barnes

# CHAPTER 9

# PATIENT STORIES

For this chapter, six of Holisticare's patients have told their stories in their own words. I asked them to talk about what caused their issues in the first place, how the issues affected their lives, their experience of treatment and the myofascial release approach, and finally what differences they have found day to day.

I have included these in my book in the hope that their stories will inspire you to look for help for your own problems, and that they will give you hope for a pain-free future. Of course, the focus of their treatment is myofascial release, and I do think that is the best approach that I have come across. But there are many different techniques available and if you can find a therapist and treatment that suit you, please do keep trying to find the solution to your pain.

I have added my notes at the end of each story to explain some of the changes that each patient went through, and to relate these changes to what you have read in the rest of this book. I hope that you find it helpful to read what other people have been through. If you have any questions about their stories or my comments, please do contact me through the Holisticare website. I am always happy to talk about what we do and how it works.

## Michaela V

In April 2005 I was running two very successful businesses, had two young children and had completed the London Marathon. I ran the 26 miles in five hours, I then completed the Moonwalk in June walking the 26 miles through the night around central London. I was the fittest I had ever been, and I felt amazing.

Just two short months later, after waking up with numbness in my left foot, which then graduated up to my knee, I was told that my life would never be the same again. I would be paralysed from the neck down because of a spinal cord tumour (an ependymoma).

In the September I had 14 hours of surgery to remove the tumour and then six weeks of radiotherapy. My tumour was so rare that my neurosurgeon had only heard of a few people in the world who had this type and none of them had walked again. The expectation was that I would be paralysed from the neck down.

I just couldn't comprehend how I could go from being this fit, active, successful businesswoman, wife, and mum with two young children to profoundly disabled in just days.

Life was a rollercoaster for many years after the surgery; I had to relearn every task, every physical movement. I had to work out how to get dressed, how to walk upstairs, how to keep my shoes on (if you don't have a lot of feeling in your feet, it's tricky!). Learning to drive again was amazing, thank heavens for automatic cars.
It was about eight months after the operation that I was able to drive to collect my children from school on my own… what an incredible feeling that was.

But the days when it was all too much just getting the children up and off to school were very frequent and I would often crawl on my hands and knees to the sofa as they left for school and stay there until 3 pm when they came home, as I was exhausted.

Sadly, I had to take the decision to sell one of my businesses as it was all too much for me to deal with. The care of the second was handed over to a team of managers, as I was not able to work.

For nine years I used a wheelchair and walking sticks and took 72 tablets of Oxycontin a day to stand up – the pain was so bad.

Then in 2014 someone drove into the back of my car. For anyone else it would have been a small shunt, but for me the whiplash injury to my spine took me right back to square one. The doctors couldn't operate on my back again and told me there was nothing more they could do.

At this point trying to deal with being a single mum and then juggling my own complex health needs, the incredible tiredness that I battled with daily, and the wall of pain was too much. I realised that conventional medicine was not treating me as a whole body but just focussing on different aspects of my health, so I started exploring alternative options.

Gentle Pilates with a qualified and experienced physio helped, as did gentle yoga. I am also a fan of acupuncture to help my energy levels.

I then heard about myofascial release and Nikki and the team at Holisticare. I was very dubious, to be honest it sounded a bit weird and how could that help me? But the gentle treatment has been a big part of my recovery and is important to maintenance of my health.

Even from that first treatment I could feel the tension lifting off my back. The process didn't hurt, which was very unusual, as every time I had a normal massage or other treatment it would be more painful and leave me wiped out for days. It was like someone was lifting bricks off my back. My posture improved after my first one-hour session, and I was literally walking taller. I even had to alter the mirror in the car to drive home as I sat higher in the car seat! Over time my body has become more awake, and the messages now seem to get through to my legs and feet so much faster. My body is literally waking up. My balance has also improved, which means that practical things like getting dressed in the morning are now much easier, I don't have to hold on to the wall all the time.

However, the biggest change for me is in my pain levels and myofascial release is something I would recommend everyone to try if they have pain. It's not magic so it will take a few sessions, but you feel the benefits immediately and for the weeks after. My back problems are major, so I now view a monthly myofascial release treatment as part of my maintenance programme to keep me well, healthy and walking.

I no longer use a wheelchair or a stick or take any painkillers and I am confident that the myofascial release is all part of the solution, keeping me well and functioning to the very best of my ability. For me, that means being as pain-free as possible so I can live my life and do what I want to do!

## Notes from the author

Michaela realised that she had to take responsibility for her recovery and be pro-active about finding treatments that worked for her. This made the difference between accepting what she was told and living with the pain and disability, and now being able to live the life that she wants. Not all patients with this condition will have the same outcome, but I think that most would see some benefit from her approach.

The myofascial release treatment was able to gently release scar tissue and restrictions that had been affecting her nerves. This reduced her pain and gave her more control of her muscles. Michaela will always need to manage her symptoms, but she has now found a way of doing this on a regular basis.

## Anna H

I was first diagnosed with rheumatoid arthritis (RA) in my very early twenties. The pain and inflammation started in my hands and feet in the mornings initially but wore off after around 20 minutes or so of moving around. One morning I woke up and couldn't straighten my arm, which is when I thought it was time to see a doctor. I was referred to a well reputed rheumatologist in Harley St and confirmed as having seronegative RA. Low doses of non-steroidal anti-inflammatory drugs (NSAIDs) did little to help, and within a couple of years, the 'flare ups' were so severe that I could barely put one foot in front of the other. The road to recovery has not only been long and winding, but an expensive one too.

Traditional medication, apart from high doses of steroids back then, did little to help, so I started investing in myself. Alternative therapies offered short term pain relief; reflexology, massage, sports massage, osteopathy, physiotherapy, chiropractors, reiki, and acupuncture all played a valuable part. I was fortunate to have supportive parents that helped fund the never-ending quest to be pain free. Elimination diets seemed to be useful but were too hard to maintain and not well controlled, meaning I was never entirely sure what caused what. Nothing shifted it entirely, despite claims from some that they could.

I went through some very, very dark patches mentally, not knowing where I would end up. Needing care? Unable to hold down a job? Maybe needing a wheelchair? All terrifying at such an early age, or indeed at any age. Lifestyle played a big part, and I was in denial of the disease. I worked long hours in the West End in advertising, sitting at a PC for hours. Late nights, too much partying and not enough sleep in defiance only compounded the problem.

Fast forward almost 30 years, I am virtually medication free and almost entirely pain-free, almost all the time. To what do I attribute that? Many things: predominantly gut health, good quality organic food, great sleep, mindful meditation, cold showers and movement – and learning to cope with the stressors in life.

I truly believe all played and continue to play a valuable role. But, most importantly, stumbling across Nikki and the Holisticare team was very much the icing on the cake.

Of all the pains throughout the body, the one that was constantly inescapable, regardless of how other joints were faring, was the pain in my neck. I had long since changed opinions on intense 'sports' type massages; it felt counter intuitive to imagine that something so painful could be doing any good. If anything, I recoiled and tensed up, shying away from the pressure.

Nikki taught me that to gently coerce the myofascial tissue into releasing was a far superior method in getting everything else to relax, a bit like taking off tights that are too small. It's true and it really works.

I can honestly say that after each treatment, I leave with freer movement in my neck than the time before and, genuinely, with no pain. Nikki is so knowledgeable, a master in her craft, and an all-round bloomin' nice person. I can't recommend her highly enough.

### *Notes from the author*

Anna's condition is not one that will be 'cured', but she has found ways to be able to keep it under control. The focus of this is working with her body, rather than against it, so her symptoms do not build up in the way that they used to.

The myofascial release treatment helps to control the compensations for the joint damage – many of the symptoms from arthritis arise from the tension surrounding the joint. This is the body's way of compensating for the underlying joint damage. Myofascial release takes the pressure off joint, making it easier to manage symptoms. In Anna's case, the combination of approaches is enabling her to live the life that she wants to.

## Toby A

Earlier this year I started to notice some problems with my left shoulder and upper arm. I don't recall injuring it but gradually the shoulder was becoming tighter to the extent that eventually I could no longer lift my left arm much over 90 degrees.

In addition, if I moved my arm up quickly, I would get a pain in my upper arm. As I got into the car and extended my arm to put my bag onto the passenger seat, I would get the pain and my arm would seem to 'fail' and lose strength and drop down.

I tried getting massages and tried all sorts of heat lotions and gels, but nothing seemed to resolve the problems.

After some months, I saw Nikki Robinson at a networking event, and she suggested that I visit her practice. She explained the concepts of myofascial release and, while admittedly somewhat sceptical, I decided it was worth trying.

On my first visit to see Nikki, she checked the alignment of my pelvis and then gently reset it. I was amazed how such gentle pressure could have such a beneficial effect. She taught me about the psoas muscles and gave me some simple exercises to do at home to help improve them so that my whole body could start working better.

By the end of the second session with Nikki, I was able to lift my arm much higher, and over the next two sessions, she worked on and around my shoulder and upper arm, still just using gentle pressure. Within a couple of weeks, I was able to lift my left arm right up and there is now virtually no difference in the range of my left and right.

The whole experience of the treatment that I received from Nikki was pleasant and involved no pain at all. She carefully explained everything that she was doing and the reasons behind it as well as the exercises that she gave me to do at home.

Several weeks later and I am pleased to say that I have none of the issues that I had previously – I can extend my arm while holding weight and do things like put my bag on the passenger seat of the car again.

Needless to say, I am no longer sceptical – indeed I am amazed at the fantastic and long-lasting results from such a gentle therapy, and I have no hesitation in recommending Nikki and Holisticare.

### *Notes from the author*

The pain in Toby's shoulder was probably caused by inflammation linked to restrictions elsewhere in his body. These build up gradually over time, until your body can no longer compensate for them. Correcting his pelvic alignment early in the treatment took a lot of the stress out of his system. His body was then able to start to reduce the inflammation, which together with more localised treatment, reduced his pain and improved the range of movement.

### Nick M

I'm one of those people who has suffered through most of my middle and later life with aches and pains in my lower back and down my legs/in my knees. I was never particularly sure of the cause, although I expect being overweight and short on exercise would have been contributory factors. I have had varying degrees of pain and they impacted upon me in different ways at different times. Typically, my back would be sore when I got out of bed in the morning, my knees and other parts of my legs would ache from time to time, sciatica was certainly a regular feature and I was conscious that stretching, especially in bed, increasingly resulted in my calf going into cramp. My daughter had benefited from treatment with Nikki and that spurred me on to see what could be done.

The experience of most treatments was not, it's fair to say, a rapid 'lightening flash' healing one, nor did they produce instant or everlasting cures necessarily. What they did do was give me a sense of my body and the relationships between its various parts (muscles I guess in the main). I had not understood previously how pain in one part could be being caused by something going on elsewhere. I also became aware that I am not a naturally 'feeling' person. I've been asked by Ali (one of the therapists at Holisticare) how such and such felt – did I feel anything? Or how did that feel? And the answer was *"No, not really"* or *"Yes, fine"*. However, what I soon learnt was that over time, and generally a day or two after each session, the impact would work through and I would genuinely feel better – less pain, looser, more easily able to move without sciatic pain and, lo and behold, my back didn't hurt in the morning! For her part, Ali tried to get more out of me but accepted in the end that I couldn't describe what was going on inside because I couldn't actually tell anything was going on inside! But it clearly was.

My attendance at Holisticare has been off and on over the five years since I first started. I've tended to come and go as the need arose. As things have got better for me, so I have stopped until something else happened. Most recently in autumn 2021, after a long spell of non-attendance, I fell (stupidly) off a ladder and wrenched the muscles in my upper right arm trying to grab hold of a support to prevent the fall. Happily, I've never dislocated my shoulder, but when I fell, the pain was so excruciating that this was what I thought I must have done. Once the immediate pain wore off, I was left with continual aching and very restricted movement, and I couldn't lie on my right side in bed. I suffered for a few weeks thinking it would get better until I remembered Holisticare! From November through to just before Christmas, I had weekly sessions that proved to be an almost immediate salve. I don't know what she did, but *"miracle hands"* sorted me out – the pain receded quite quickly, and I got back my movement. The full healing took a bit longer, but it was completely bearable in the aftermath of the treatment.

I'm currently attending regularly for maintenance sessions rather than to deal with a particular issue. That's been helpful and has encouraged me to mentally record what is going on as I live my life – when I go for a walk, does it hurt anywhere and if so, where? Then I can relay the experience with more clarity so that more targeted treatment is, I presume, possible. I know that treatments aren't everlasting and so I hope that this regular attention approach will help to keep me on, or at least closer to the 'straight and narrow'.

## Notes from the author

Nick's description of having difficulty feeling the changes during treatment is a common one and, as he demonstrates, you do not need to be able to feel what is happening to benefit from the treatment. Although receiving regular treatments does tend to make it easier to feel, not everyone gets there. It is worth persevering with focusing on what is occurring, though, as the ability to perceive these subtle changes makes it much easier to follow your body and prevent problems day to day.

## Deborah H

Nikki Robinson is an amazing myofascial release therapist. She also has a wonderful team who work at Holisticare.

Just to give you a little bit of my history, I am 67 years old and have run a riding school for the past 40 years. So, I like to consider myself a fairly active person, as I still run the riding school to this day.

About 30 years ago I fell down some stairs, landing on my coccyx. This was extremely painful, and I couldn't ride for the next six weeks. However, it seemed to clear up, and I resumed riding and carried on as normal.

Approximately seven years ago I developed a condition called coccydynia which I believe was caused by my fall all those years ago. It is an extremely painful condition which becomes aggravated when sitting down. What was even more painful, believe it or not, was trying to stand up. The pain of my coccyx unwinding when I got out of a chair or the car was unbelievable and it made me look like a very old person! I tried various treatments which sadly didn't work. Three years running I had a steroid injection into my coccyx. Yes, the injections did take the pain away, but the pain always returned within a year.

I then met the wonderful Nikki Robinson who told me about myofascial release. As I was still in pain and going nowhere fast, I felt I had nothing to lose but to try myofascial release. Before having my first treatment, Nikki asked me lots of questions about my general health in the past. Without realising it at the time, my answers helped influence how she treated me. Her hands-on approach really worked and made a huge difference. There is no pushing, pulling, twisting, just firm pressure. I don't know how she does it, but she always finds the right spot. I could literally feel the change under her hands. I remember Nikki saying she treats the cause and not the symptoms and I really took that on board. I'm delighted to say I can now sit very comfortably anywhere and go for long drives in my car without pain. I am a different person thanks to the treatment at Holisticare.

Unfortunately I had another accident in May last year, just after lockdown. It happened to be our first day back and I was helping one of our riders mount his horse. Unexpectedly, I fell off our mounting ramp and landed heavily onto concrete. I severely damaged my right shoulder, so once again, I went to Holisticare. With their warm welcome, professional approach and wonderful hands my shoulder is well on the mend. In fact, I am not receiving any treatment now as they helped me so much and I continued with the exercises they suggested. Myofascial release is phenomenal, and I could not recommend it more.

Thank you to Nikki, your team and Holisticare for literally changing my life for the better.

### Notes from the author

I am so glad that myofascial release treatment was able to break Deborah's pain cycle.

Unfortunately, steroid injections often only have a limited effect, and they only treat the symptoms, not the cause. It is likely that Deborah had scar tissue and restrictions around her coccyx from the original fall, which then developed into the very painful inflammation.

Now she knows about our treatment, any further injuries can be treated straight away, so they don't turn into a chronic condition in the future.

## Sarah H

The car accident itself had seemed such a minor thing until the next day, and the day after that, when my shoulders and neck began to seize up. And every day after that the screws just seemed to tighten until my body was full of pain, my neck would go into a spasm, and I would get stuck where I was.

My GP prescribed strong painkillers that made me too drowsy and woozy to do anything when I took them, which really wasn't any kind of solution. The car insurance organised some physiotherapy sessions, but after the allotted six, I still couldn't move my head properly, do any sports, lift anything heavier than a kettle, and I couldn't work.

The physio said I just needed to try exercising for 5 minutes a day and build up. So, dutifully, the next day I did 5 gentle minutes of warm up exercises and spent the next three days unable to get out of bed.

Eventually, after I had received thirty sessions of physiotherapy, the insurance company needed to settle before court proceedings, and a specialist from Harley Street was brought in. He examined me, read the reports, and told me that it was time, time for me to accept that I had lost, and would never regain, 40% of the movement in my neck.

There would be no more sports, my reflexology business was gone, I couldn't dig, or push a lawnmower in my beloved garden. I couldn't even do the simplest things like put out my own wheelie bin! And my pain, as well as being in my neck, head, shoulders and back, had now progressed into carpal tunnel in both hands.

The financial compensation that I received when the case was settled was no compensation at all for these loses. My life looked nothing like the one that I had before that silly accident. I lived with pain and frustration, and no-one seemed to understand that taking tablets was not going to be a long term (if any term) solution for me.

It was over a decade later when I was introduced to Nikki at a meeting, I had never heard of myofascial technique, I was sceptical, but when we met again, I thought it was something worth trying.

I personally found it challenging to fill in the forms – but is facing up to things ever pretty? The initial session made me feel a lot more comfortable, hopeful even. Nikki was so calm and gentle, she didn't tell me what I should be doing, or make me feel like my issues were too big for the clinic or too small to bother with.

With no expectation I had a session. It felt good, relaxing, but I didn't understand why there was no pushing, prodding, pulling or cracking. What were they doing?

After a few weekly sessions my posture had changed, people were commenting that I was looking well, for the first time in over a decade my pain had decreased to such an extent that I could hold my head up. I could actually look forward for hours at a time! When you have spent so long looking at the floor because it's too painful to lift your head, let me tell you, everything looks amazing!

Something else that I noticed from the treatments actually showed itself in my sessions with my counsellor. After many years of talking therapies for life limiting phobias, despite many hours of talking and processing, I still found it extremely hard to process the emotions and therefore free myself from my deep-seated issues.

It was not instantaneous, but gradually I found a new willingness to open myself to emotional healing. Within a year my inner life was also considerably healthier. My therapist has noticed a marked change in me and my ability to manage my condition.

I tell people about Nikki and her team all the time. I simply say if you are in pain, don't be afraid to go to Holisticare, that's what I did.

I am now enjoying yoga, and long walks (I did a 60km walk for charity not too long ago). And bliss – I can work in my garden. Sometimes if I haven't been to the clinic in a couple of months, and I have been forgetting to do my exercises, the headaches, aches, and pain start to creep back. That's enough of a reminder for me to start looking after myself again, and to make an appointment at Holisticare.

### *Notes from the author*

We see so many people who end up with long-term problems from a relatively minor incident. This is because throughout your life, everything that happens to you and your body is potentially recorded in your fascial system. These create restrictions and holding patterns (long-term tension held within an area or areas of your body), that are constantly affecting your ability to adapt to life and need to be compensated for. We are very good at doing this and can often mask things for a long time.

But then the minor car crash, trip or accident can stir up all the old issues, as well as creating new ones, and you are feeling everything that your body has been compensating for. As well as being very painful and distressing, it can also impact on the recovery of the latest injury. Myofascial release treatment works with your whole body, regardless of the chronological order of the symptoms, so you are able to start to release old and new restrictions and your body can heal properly.

The mind-body connection has the potential to affect all aspects of mental health and everybody's response to the treatment will be different. But I have seen many examples of changes in my patients since I have been using myofascial release.

The form that Sarah refers to is for new patients at Holisticare, in particular the sections about your past medical history and the history of your present condition. Patients who have a complex history may find it hard to document everything in one place.

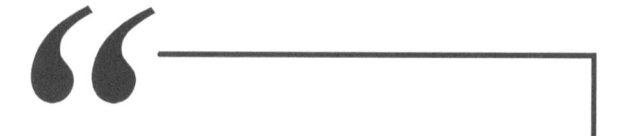

> *What if it could be easy?*
>
> John F. Barnes

# CHAPTER 10

# ONGOING HELP

There are growing numbers of therapists being trained in John Barnes's myofascial release in the US and the UK, and they will all have differing backgrounds and amounts of experience. However, if they are following the principles of this technique, you should be able to be confident that they will follow your body during the treatment, without forcing anything.

To find a therapist near you in the UK, I can recommend looking on the *"Find a Practitioner"* page on the Myofascial Release UK website: myofascialrelease.uk.

My specialist myofascial release practice is called Holisticare. We are based on a working farm on the Hertfordshire / Essex border in England.
All our therapists are trained in John Barnes's myofascial release, and our patients travel to us from all over the UK and Europe to receive our expert treatment.
If you would like more information, please have a look at our website: www.holisticare.co.uk.

## Holisticare

**HOLISTICARE**

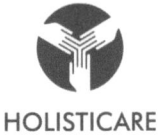

Holisticare is a centre of excellence and expertise, providing hope to people who think they can't be helped, in a safe, caring, and relaxed environment.

At Holisticare, we specialise in John F. Barnes myofascial release. John Barnes is the American physiotherapist who developed this *"innovative and highly effective whole-body approach for evaluation and treatment."*

Our patient-centred approach means that every session is different, depending on the needs of that patient on that day. This is determined by what the therapist and patient feel and communicate to each other during the treatment. Our expertise and experience allow us to successfully work with people who have tried everything else and have not seen any improvement in their condition.

Patients at Holisticare are always seen at their booked appointment time; we pride ourselves on not keeping you waiting.

We pride ourselves on providing our patients with a service that comes from the heart. We feel that therapy doesn't only happen on the treatment couch but in all our interactions with our patients.

Our mission is to be recognised as the foremost provider of myofascial release, providing expert treatment in a compassionate, caring manner.

## The Let it Go Programme

The Let it Go Programme is designed to allow the patient to focus on their own physical and emotional needs away from the distractions and stresses of everyday life.

With the choice of 3 days, 1 week or 2 weeks, giving you 3 hours of treatment per day, this programme is designed to help you to make long-lasting changes to your life.

If you would like to find out more, please have a look at our website: www.holisticare.co.uk.

## Freedom From Pain and Tension – online programme

Juggling the demands of family and work, even if you are not living with chronic pain, can be extremely challenging. Taking some time out for yourself to relax, release and renew will benefit your health and well-being, enabling you to meet those demands calmly and under control.

The aim of the Freedom From Pain & Tension programme is to teach you how to follow your body so you can prevent and reduce the pain that so many people live with.

The programme is made up of the following modules, each divided into several techniques. By the end of the programme, you will have the tools to treat all areas of your body, with a much greater understanding of why your symptoms occur.

- *Module 1:* Your neck and upper back
- *Module 2:* Your lower back
- *Module 3:* Your legs
- *Module 4:* Your arms
- *Module 5:* Your hands and feet
- *Module 6:* Your head and face

Each module includes:

- Information about your body and how it works.
- Four self-treatment techniques on video and PDF.
- Relaxation/visualisation audio.

You will have lifetime access to all the modules when you log in, allowing you to work through the programme at a time and pace to suit your schedule and on any device.

If you would like to sign up, simply go to this website: https://holisticare.systeme.io/freedom-full

## Mailing list

To receive updates, tips and special offers from Holisticare, please email info@holisticare.co.uk

## Pain-Free Horse Riding

My first book, Pain-Free Horse Riding, is a practical guide for horse riders of all abilities and disciplines to show them how to reduce and prevent pain. It has been published in the UK and North America and is available worldwide as an e-book.

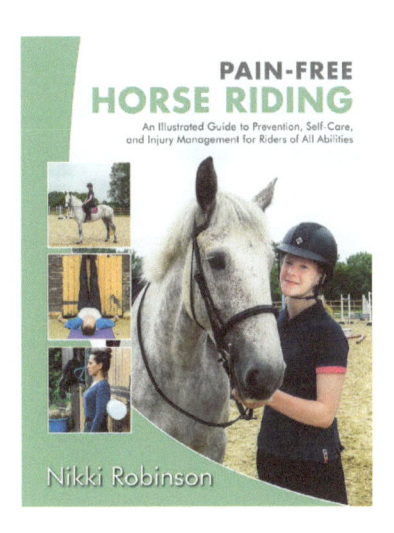

You can order your copy from www.painfreehorseriding.com.

## Get in touch

www.facebook.com/HolisticareMFR

www.holisticare.co.uk

info@holisticare.co.uk

# ACKNOWLEDGMENTS

Huge thanks and appreciation to my longsuffering family – Pete, Freddy, Joey, and Katie, who put up with me having bright ideas! And to Katie for allowing me to use her as a model again.

Also, thanks to the amazing team at Holisticare and my lovely patients for their encouragement and making me believe that I was capable of putting my passion into words.

Thank you to Ellie for your support and guidance, and holding me accountable, to Danielle for your skill in editing and proof-reading, and to Lois for your amazing cover design.

Sarah the photographer and Gabrielle the illustrator: you are very talented, and it is always a pleasure to work with both of you.

Nikki from The Printsave Group, thank you as always for your professionalism and for making this book look great.

I really appreciate the lovely words written by John F. Barnes in the Foreword.

Thank you to Sally and Jean for patiently reading through what I had written and giving great feedback, and to my friends and networking buddies for their support and introductions.

This book wouldn't be the same without the words from my patients about their experiences. Thank you all so much for your generosity and for being part of this book.

# BIBLIOGRAPHY

Davis, C. M. *"Integrative Therapies in Rehabilitation."* Thorofare, NJ Slack, 2017.

Duncan, R. *"Myofascial Release."* Leeds, UK: Human Kinetics, 2014.

EDHS.info. *"Understanding Ehlers-Danlos Syndrome Hypermobility-Type and Joint Hypermobility Syndrome."* EDS-H & JHS. Last updated 2013, accessed 16 June 2018. https://www.edhs.info/what-is-eds-h.

Liptan G. *"The FibroManual."* New York: Ballantine Books, 2016.

Pollack, G. H. *"The Fourth Phase of Water."* Seattle, WA: Ebner and Sons, 2013.

Sling the Mesh. *"What Is the Campaign About?"* WordPress. N.d., accessed 16 June 2018. https://slingthemesh.wordpress.com/.

Travell, J., D. Simons, and L. Simons. *"Myofascial Pain and Dysfunction: The Trigger Point Manual."* 2nd ed. 2 vols. Baltimore, MD: Lippincott Williams and Williams, 1999.

# GLOSSARY

*Achilles tendon:* the tendon that attaches your calf muscle to your heel bone.

*Acute injury or pain:* happens suddenly, usually as a result of an injury.

*Adrenal glands:* small, triangular-shaped glands located on the top of your kidneys. They produce hormones that help to regulate essential functions in your body such as metabolism, immune system, blood pressure and response to stress.

*Adrenalin:* a hormone produced by the adrenaline glands that prepare your body for 'fight or flight'.

*Arthritis:* a condition that causes pain and swelling in joints.

*Auto-immune disorder:* diseases that occur when the body's natural defence system can't tell the difference between your own cells and foreign cells, causing the body to mistakenly attack normal cells.

*Autonomic nervous system:* the part of your nervous system that regulates bodily functions that are out of your conscious control, such as digestion, respiration, and heart rate.

*Biotensegrity:* the relationship between every part of an organism and the mechanical system that integrates them into a complete functional unit.

*Blood pressure:* a reading of the pressure created in your blood vessels when your heart beats, and the pressure when your heart rests between beats.

*Bursitis:* inflammation of the bursa (fluid-filled sacks that cushion your joints).

*Cardiovascular system:* your heart and blood system that supplies your body with oxygen and nutrients.

*Carpal tunnel syndrome:* pressure on a nerve in your wrist which causes pain, numbness and tingling in your hand and fingers.

*Cartilage:* tough, flexible tissue that acts as a shock absorber and protection for bony ends in your joints.

*Chronic:* a disease or pain that lasts for a long time or is recurring.

*Collagen:* a protein produced by your body that forms part of the structure and function of all your connective tissue.

*Cortisol:* a stress hormonal produced by your adrenal glands.

*COVID-19:* an infectious disease caused by the SARS-CoV-2 virus.

*Digestive system:* made up of the digestive tract and other organs that help the body break down and absorb food.

*Dislocation:* an injury that occurs when the bones in a joint are forced out of place.

*Elastin:* a very stretchy protein that forms part of your connective tissue.

*Endorphins:* hormones produced by the pituitary gland in the brain that block the perception of pain and increase feelings of well-being.

*Fascia:* the continuous tissue that connects every cell of your body.

*Fibromyalgia:* a chronic condition that typically causes fatigue and pain all over the body.

*Fractal:* a complex shape that consists of infinitely repeating patterns.

*Fracture:* a break in a bone.

*Frozen shoulder:* inflammation of the joint capsule in the shoulder, causing pain and stiffness.

*Golfer's elbow:* inflammation of the tendon on the inside of your elbow.

*Ground substance:* a gel-like substance that fills all the spaces between cells and connective tissue fibres in your body.

*Hydration:* the process of absorbing water into your body.

*Hypermobility:* a syndrome where some or all of a person's joints have an unusually large range of movement.

*Inflammation:* part of your body's immune response, to aid healing or to fight harmful agents.

*Intervertebral discs:* cushions of fibro-cartilage between each vertebra that act as separators and shock absorbers.

*Ligaments:* fibrous connective tissue that attaches bone to bone.

*Long COVID:* signs and symptoms that develop during or after COVID-19 infection and last longer than 12 weeks.

*Lymph:* the fluid that flows through the lymphatic system.

*Lymphatic system:* a network of tissues, vessels and organs that work together to move lymph back into your bloodstream.

*Myalgic encephalomyelitis (ME):* a long-term condition that causes persistent fatigue, also called chronic fatigue syndrome.

*Myofascial release:* a gentle hands-on treatment that enables restrictions in your body to be released.

*Neurological system:* your nervous system, consisting of your brain, spinal cord, and network of nerves.

*Osteophytes:* a smooth, bony lump that grows off a bone.

*Parasympathetic nervous system:* a network of nerves that help your body to rest and relax.

*Patella:* your kneecap.

*Pelvic floor:* a sling of muscles at the bottom of your pelvis that support your pelvic organs.

*Physiotherapy:* helps people affected by injury, illness or disability through movement and exercise, manual therapy, education, and advice.

*Plantar fasciitis:* inflammation of the membrane on the soles of your feet.

*Prolapse:* a condition in which organs fall down or slip out of place.

*Psoas muscles:* a pair of muscles that support your lower back and flex your hips.

*Psychological:* related to the mental and emotional state of a person.

*Quadriceps muscles:* your thigh muscles.

*Repetitive strain injury:* injury caused by repeated use of a body part.

*Respiratory system:* the organs and other parts of your body involved in breathing.

*Rotator cuff:* a group of muscles and tendons that hold the shoulder joint in place and allow you to move your arm and shoulder.

*Sciatica:* pain that travels along the path of the sciatic nerve – from your back, through your buttocks and down the back of your leg.

*Sympathetic nervous system:* a network of nerves that respond to dangerous or stressful situations.

*Tendonitis:* inflammation of a tendon.

*Tendons:* bands of connective tissue that connect muscles to bones.

*Tennis elbow:* inflammation of the tendons on the outside of your elbow.

*Tensegrity:* a structure with a balance between compression and distraction forces.

*Thixotropic:* a property of some gels or fluids that change state depending on temperature and applied stress.

# INDEX

## Symbols
"-Itis", 44, 52, 55

## A
anatomy, 11
anti-inflammatory response stimulation, 80
autonomic nervous system, **15**, 16, 91, 141
    parasympathetic nervous system, **16**, 143
    sympathetic nervous system, **16**, 17, 19, 23, 144

## B
back pain, 17, **36**, 38, 41, 49, 56, 69, 77
    psoas muscles, **17**, 37, 88, 89, 81, 144
    psoas release with ball, 89
    red flag symptoms, 36
    spine release with foam roller, 91
Barnes, John F, **1**, 4, 79, 111, 117, 133, 137. *See also* mayofascial release
biotensegrity, **11**, 12, 13, 14, 141.
*See also* fascia
Blu Tack, 112
body scan, 80
body's reaction to injury, 15
    emotional response, 18
    physical response, 15
    self-help, 21-24
body abnormalities, 50
breath, holding, 62
    diaphragm release, 87
breathing, **59**, 60-63, 75, 80, 87, 92, 99. *See also* self-help for posture and symptom reduction
    diaphragm, 23, 60, 61, 62, 87, 88
    diaphragmatic, 61, 62
    effects of wrong, 60
    problems, 59, 60
    proper way of, 60, 61, 62
buttocks release with ball, 96

## C
calf release with a ball, 97
chronic obstructive pulmonary disease (COPD), 59
concussion, 24, 25. *See also* body's reaction to injury

connective tissue, 1, 9, 40, 83, 111, 117, 142, 143, 144. *See* fascia

consciousness, altered state of,, 18. *See also* body's reaction to injury

constructive rest position, 91, 92

contract/relax method, 81, 82, 95

    for arms, 81

    for hips, 95

    for lower legs, 82

COPD, 59. *See* chronic obstructive pulmonary disease (COPD)

COVID, 47, 48, 56, 142, 143. *See also* Long COVID

# D

diaphragm, 23, 60, 61, 62, 87, 88. *See also* breathing

    breathing, 59, 60, 61, 62, 63, 75, 80, 87, 92, 99

    release, 87

direct psoas release, 37, 89

# E

EDS, 40, 139. *See* Ehlers-Danlos syndrome

Ehlers-Danlos syndrome (EDS), 40, 139

elbow pain and stiffness, 44

    elbow release, 98

    tension in back and neck, 30

# F

falls, 22, 23, 25, 30

    how to help yourself after a,, 23

fascia, 1, 7, 9, 10, 11, 13, 14, 15, 19, 52, 116, 117, 142

    biotensegrity, 11, 12, 13, 14, 141

    fascial network, 10, 15, 22, 55, 113

    in healthy conditions, 10

    in trauma, 10

    myofascial architecture, 13, 14

    parts of, 10

    tensegrity model, 11

fascial network, 10, 15, 22, 55, 113. *See also* fascia function

fascial system, 10, 12, 13, 18, 19, 20, 22, 30, 33, 111, 113. *See also* mayofascial release

fibromyalgia, 20, 38, 39, 56, 91, 142

    constructive rest position, 92

fight-or-flight muscle, 17. *See* psoas muscle

finger pulls, 102

foam roller, 83, 87, 88, 90, 91, 93, 94, 95

foot release with ball, 104

freeze response, 17, 60. *See also* body's reaction to injury frozen memory and traumas, 18. *See also* body's reaction to injury

Fuller, Buckminster, 11

## G

golfer's elbow, 45, 55, 98, 142. *See also* elbow pain and stiffness

Guimberteau, Dr, Jean-Claude, 10, 13, 14

## H

hamstring release, 93

hand and wrist pain and stiffness, 44

    finger pulls, 102

    hand-on-ball release, 102

healing crisis, 115, 116, 117. *See also* mayofascial release

hip, 17, 29, 46, 72, 73, 77, 87, 88, 93, 94, 95, 98, 144

hip pain and stiffness, 46

    hamstring release, 93

    IT band release with roller, 94, 95

hypermobility syndrome, 40, 139

    need for therapist's assessment, 40

## I

immobility response, 17, 18. *See also* body's reaction to injury

inflammation, 10, 19, 28, 31, 32, 33, 38, 44, 45, 46, 48, 51, 52, 55, 56, 64, 67, 99, 111, 141, 142, 143, 144

internal scarring, 53, 54

intervertebral discs, 37, 143

IT band release with roller, 94, 95

## J

joint degeneration, 50. *See* osteoarthritis

joint pain and stiffness, 44

joint replacement, 47

## K

Kegel, Arnold, 42

Kegel exercises, 42

knee pain and stiffness, 46

## L

lifting safely, 71, 72, 73, 77. *See also* working safely

Liptan, Ginevra, 138

Long COVID, 47, 48, 143. *See also* COVID

lower back, 37, 75, 88, 91, 93, 144

    psoas release, 37, 98

thigh release, 92-95

buttocks release with ball, 96

# M

moderate-intensity exercise, 1, 4, 79, 111, 117, 133, 137

muscles, 7, 8, 9, 12, 16, 17, 22, 30, 31, 35, 36, 37, 39, 41, 42, 43, 45, 46, 47, 49, 51, 52, 53, 55, 58, 60, 62, 64, 67, 71, 74, 79, 83, 85, 86, 88, 89, 91, 92, 93, 94, 143, 144

myofascial architecture, 13, 14. *See also* fascia

myofascial release, 1, 4, 35, 38, 39, 45, 48, 50, 54, 56, 67, 79, 109, 111, 112, 113, 115, 117, 131, 133, 134, 139, 143

    assessment, 35, 36, 79, 113

    healing crisis, 115, 116, 117

    therapists, 3, 112, 133

    thixotropic response, 111, 112, 144

    treatment, 39, 48, 50, 112, 113, 114

    unwinding, 116, 117

# N

National Health Service in England (NHS England), 47, 56

neck pain, 49, 50

neck release with ball, 85, 86

NHS England, 47, 56. *See* National Health Service in England (NHS England)

# O

osteoarthritis, 50

    muscle strengthening exercises, 51

    regular movement, 51

osteophytes, 51, 143

# P

pain, **27**, 28, 29, 30, 36, 39, 44, 45, 46, 49. *See also* body's reaction to injury

    chronic pain, 20, 27, 28, 29, 33, 48, 54, 134

    cycle, 28, 29

    medication, 5, 29

panic attack, 20, 21, 22, 25

parasympathetic nervous system, 16, 143

pelvic floor, , 41, 42, 43, 46, 143

pelvis, 6, 7, 8, 17, 39, 41, 42, 45, 46, 52, 55, 87, 88, 89, 143

    alignment, 6, 7, 8, 39, 42, 45, 46, 52

    floor exercises, 42

    wonky, 42

plantar fascia, 52

plantar fasciitis, 33, 52, 104, 143

    foot release with ball, 104

    self-treatment, 79, 104

post lean, 100, 101

postural problems, 68

postural problems by, 68. *See also* self-help for posture and symptom reduction

    carrying shopping, 69

    computer work, 66, 75, 76

    driving, , 68

    gardening, 66, 73, 74

    holding phone between ear and shoulder, 76

    looking after babies and children, 77

    messaging, 76

    staying in same position, 66, 69, 75

    using laptops, 76

    walking dog, 68

psoas muscle, 17, 37, 88, 89, 81, 144

    release in standing, 89

    psoas release with ball, 89

    release with chair, 90

# Q

quadriceps exercises, 46, 92

# R

recovering from hard day, 98

repetitive strain injury (RSI), 52, 53, 56, 144

    trigger identification, 53

Romanesco cauliflower, 13

rotated pelvis, 7, 8, 46, 55

    strain on body by, 46

rounded shoulders, 9, 21, 49, 68, 99, 101

    shoulder stretch with upright post, 101

RSI, 52, 53, 56, 144. *See* repetitive strain injury (RSI)

# S

scar tissue, 11, 19, 28, 32, 39, 45, 47, 53, 54, 84, 113

    internal scarring, 53, 54

    self-treatment, 84

self-help for posture and symptom reduction, 79 - 109

    postural problem activities, 68, 69

    releasing tension, 101, 107

    stretching, 97, 112

    water intake, 44, 54, 57, 59, 69, 75, 115, 116, 142

    way of breathing, 59

shoulder, 39, 45, 49, 50, 52, 53, 55, 60, 68, 69, 72, 73, 85, 86, 99,

100, 101, 142, 144
- circles, 99
- injury, 45, 53
- rotator cuff, 53, 55, 99, 144
- rotators release, 99
- stretch with upright post, 101

shoulder circles, 99

shoulder pain and stiffness, 45

shoulders, elevated, 49, 68
- self-treatment, 1, 4, 79, 111, 117, 133, 137
- upper trapezius, 50, 86

side stretch, 87

spine release with foam roller, 90, 91

strain, 7, 8, 10, 12, 15, 31, 32, 42, 44, 46, 48, 51, 52, 53, 56, 73, 76, 77, 102, 106, 109, 117, 144
- by rotated pelvic bones, 7, 8

strengthening exercises for muscles around joint, 40, 41, 46, 51

stress cycle, 20. *See also* body's reaction to injury

stretching, 6, 31, 40, 64, 65, 66, 97, 112. *See also* body's reaction to injury
- morning stretch, 64
- reasons for feeling tight, 64
- ways to do, 64, 65, 97, 112

surgery, 1, 19, 41, 45, 47, 54

sweeping, 74

sympathetic nervous system, 16, 17, 19, 23, 144

symptoms, common, 21, 27, 35
- inflammation, 28, 31, 32
- pain, 27, 28, 29, 30, 31, 32, 33
- tension, 30, 31, 33

# T

tendonitis, 44, 46, 55, 144
- gentle movement, 56
- muscles affected by, 55
- rest, 55
- self-treatment, 79

tendons, 36, 44, 45, 49, 52, 53, 55, 144

tennis elbow, 33, 45, 144

tensegrity model, 11. *See also* fascia

tension, 7, 9, 10, 11, 17, 18, 19, 21, 23, **30**, 31, 33, 37, 38, 45, 48, 49, 50, 51, 55, 60, 63, 65, 66, 68, 69, 74, 75, 76, 79, 80, 84, 85, 87, 90, 91, 97, 99, 101, 105, 106, 107, 111, 131

tension release, 101, 107. *See also* self-help for posture and symptom reduction
- myofascial release treatment, 39, 48, 50, 67, 112, 113

thigh release, 92-95

with ball, 93
with chair, 93

thixotropic, 111, 112, 144. *See also* mayofascial release

tired legs, 98. *See also* working safely

tools, 73. *See also* working safely

trauma, 3, 10, 17, 18, 19, 23, 24, 32, 36, 38, 41, 45, 47, 48, 115, 117
    fascia in, 10, 15, 18, 19, 20, 23, 24, 32
    frozen memory and, 18

# U

unwinding, 116, 117, 128. *See also* mayofascial release

upper trapezius, 50, 86

urinary incontinence, 40, 41
    need for treatment, 42
    pelvic floor exercises, 42
    types of, 41
    water intake, 44

urinary tract infection (UTI), 58

UTI, 58. *See* urinary tract infection (UTI)

# W

water intake, 44, 54, 57, 59, 69, 75, 115, 116, 142. *See also* self-help for posture and symptom reduction
    effects of dehydration, 30, 58
    effects of more, 57
    importance of, 57
    urinary incontinence, 40, 41
    ways to increase, 59

wear and tear, 37, 50, 53, 57. *See* osteoarthritis

wheelbarrow, 73, 74

working safely, 71, 72, 73, 74, 75, 76, 77
    lifting, 71, 72, 73, 77
    recovering from hard day, 1, 4, 79, 111, 117, 133, 137
    tools, 73